Dictionary of
Childhood Health Problems

Dictionary of Childhood Health Problems

2nd Edition

Patricia Gilbert

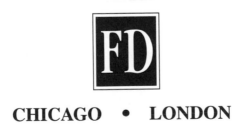

CHICAGO • LONDON

Copyright © 2000 Patricia Gilbert

All rights reserved including the right of reproduction in whole or in part in any form. For information write to:

FITZROY DEARBORN PUBLISHERS
919 North Michigan Avenue
Chicago, Illinois 60611
USA

or

FITZROY DEARBORN PUBLISHERS
310 Regent Street
London W1R 5AJ
England

British Library and Library of Congress Cataloguing in Publication Data are available.

ISBN 1-57958-213-3

First published in the USA 2000
This edition first published in the UK 2000

Contents

Acknowledgements

My thanks are due, once again, to Dr. Terry Billington for the superb work done in reading this manuscript. Her comments and suggestions have been gratefully received, but any errors are entirely my own.

I would like to thank Tony Wayte at Stanley Thorne for his ever-willing availability for discussion on the format of this second edition.

As ever, my wider thanks are due to the many children and their parents who, over the years, have allowed me into their homes and lives when problems of health have arisen.

Preface to the Second Edition

The original text covered conditions that mainly affect children over the age of 2 years; these conditions are not necessarily unknown in younger children, but they are less likely to occur before the second birthday.

There are, however, health problems that can arise solely in the younger child, such as, for example, bronchiolitis, pyloric stenosis, and roseola infantum. To provide a more complete overview of children's health problems, several of these conditions have been added to this edition. Obviously, only a selection of childhood ills can be mentioned in the space of a small volume, and the conditions added here are the ones most likely to be seen in everyday situations.

Sections on various generic symptoms, such as headaches and rashes, have also been added. Again, while this book's list of possible causes of each of these signs and symptoms is not necessarily exhaustive, the entries may provide clues as to possible underlying factors. It must be stressed, however, that children can become seriously ill in a very short space of time, and delay in obtaining medical help can be dangerous.

A short discussion on the current schedule of immunization procedures has also been added. This information is, of course, subject to change in the light of new knowledge and/or new vaccines becoming available.

It is hoped that this extended version will be of greater value to a wider range of readers who care daily for children.

Patricia Gilbert
May 1998

Preface to the First Edition

Children, as well as adults, become ill. The onset of sometimes severe, or even life-threatening, illness can occur at any time and in any place. For instance, a child may seem perfectly well when setting off for school, but by midday he or she can be burning with fever, in severe pain, or in urgent need of hospitalization.

Anyone who cares for children, and certainly those many dedicated people who spend their lives working with children, needs a basic knowledge of childhood illnesses. Knowledge of emergency treatment for a variety of conditions, information about disease prevention and the spread of infectious disease, and knowledge of the natural history of the illness are all valuable to care givers. Teachers, daycare employees, and social workers, as well as those people more intimately concerned with the care of sick children, need a quick, ready reference for unexpected events that may occur during the course of a working day. Parents and foster parents also need a readily available reference source.

It is hoped that this volume will prove of value in this context. The alphabetical arrangement facilitates rapid access to the appropriate condition. The index is also comprehensively arranged to allow for specific symptoms to lead the reader to the most likely cause of the problem.

Long-term implications as well as possible later complications are found under the appropriate headings. The emphasis is on the practical day-to-day management of the many common—and some less common—illnesses affecting children.

The conditions included here fall into two broad categories. First, the book provides discussion of relatively common conditions, those from which many children will suffer during the course of their early lives. Included are common infectious illnesses such as gastroenteritis, chicken pox, and tonsillitis, as well as such diverse conditions as bedwetting, warts, and eczema. Second, the book encompasses certain less common conditions that are important to understand in order to ensure that the affected child can be helped to lead as normal a life as is possible within the limitations of the condition. This group includes such conditions as diabetes, epilepsy, and celiac disease, as well as other possibly less well known conditions, such as Perthes disease and epidermolysis bullosa. All these conditions can be found among both schoolchildren and their younger brothers and sisters.

A glossary of some relevant medical terms has been added at the end of the book, and, where appropriate, names and addresses of self-help groups have been included at the end of each specific section.

It is hoped that this book will be a valuable "working companion" to the many people involved in the vital day-to-day care of the up-and-coming generation.

Special Features of Children's Diseases

Children are not mini-adults. They are special people in their own right with special problems and needs. These facts are probably never so obvious as when a child becomes ill.

PATTERNS OF ILLNESS

Illness, in everyone, can be broken down into five basic causative factors.

Disease (or "lack of ease") can be due to a **congenital** problem. This category includes a multitude of syndromes, more and more of which are being recognized, described, and classified with each passing week. A congenital disease is one that is present from birth, and it often has its roots in a genetic or chromosomal defect. These defects may be inherited from either parent, or they can be the result of a mutation during cell division. Examples of this type of problems can range from the serious to the relatively minor. For example, Down syndrome is the result of a chromosomal abnormality, the results of which have far-ranging effects for the child and his or her family throughout life. Another example of a congenital disorder is hemophilia, for which direct family links can often be identified. This disease affects only males, but it is passed on through the female line. As with Down syndrome, the effects of this congenital problem are felt throughout life.

Relatively minor congenital problems can also occur, such as webbing of the toes, or an extra digit on one hand. (In portraits of Anne Boleyn, look for the long sleeves that hide the sixth digit on one hand!) These latter findings are unlikely to cause any significant problems in later life, but they make a fascinating part of the study of family history.

Many congenital problems are obvious either at birth or during the first few weeks of life. With accurate diagnosis and sensitive advice and discussion, parents can be helped to come to terms with their child's congenital condition, and they can be shown ways to help their child grow to reach his or her full potential with the help of other people concerned with the care of the child—daycare staff members and teachers bringing their own special expertise.

1

Second, **infections** of all kinds play a large part in the illnesses of children. Newborn babies arrive in the world with some immunity to the infections that surround us all the time. This immunity is passed on from mother to child both prenatally and in breast milk—provided, of course, that the mother herself has contracted and overcome the specific disease or has been vaccinated against it. For example, if a mother has neither suffered an attack of measles (which might have been subclinical) nor been vaccinated, she will have no antibodies available in her body to pass on to her baby. Therefore, the baby will be susceptible to this infection, should it be met. As the baby grows and matures, immunity to infectious diseases will be gained as she or he suffers from the infections or is vaccinated against them. The process of gaining of natural immunity constitutes a large part of the experience of childhood illness.

Before they acquire active immunization against a number of infections, children can become gravely ill—sometimes with fatal results—from the so-called childhood infections. Today's children in the Western world are fortunate indeed that vaccines are available to prevent large-scale epidemics (which once occurred with monotonous regularity) of such diseases as diphtheria, polio, measles, mumps, and rubella.

However, infections such as sore throats, headaches, and runny noses still abound, and lucky is the child—and his or her parents—who escapes with only a few of these episodes in the preschool and early school years. Unfortunately, unlike childhood infections such as mumps and chicken pox, the bacteria/viruses causing the common cold undergo subtle changes every year or so. Therefore, the immunity gained one year against one specific type of cold infection is not effective against the infections occurring the following year. Thus, a seemingly endless round of upper respiratory infections persists throughout the early years of childhood.

Other more serious forms of infection, such as meningitis, are also hazards to be remembered when a child becomes ill. Immunization has recently become available against one particular form of meningitis, but there are a number of other infectious agents that can cause this serious disease.

Today's children are also fortunate that powerful antibiotics are available to fight against infectious disease. However, these drugs are usually effective only against bacterial infections (with very few exceptions). Viral infections are not helped by antibiotics.

In sum, infections of all kinds account for much of the illness that happens during the childhood years. Furthermore, in spite of modern medicines and treatments, long-term complications—and fatalities—do still occur.

Third, new growths or **tumors** cause illness in children as well as adults. Cancers of all kinds affect children, leukemia (a cancer of the blood) perhaps being the most common and best-known type of malignancy. The types of tumor encountered in childhood typically differ from adult cancers. Some kinds are similar, but there are a number of cancers that are specific to childhood, such as Wilms' tumor and retinoblastoma.

This group of illnesses must always be remembered as a possible concern when a child is ill for an unusually long time. Cancer is now second only to accidents as a cause of death among children ages 1 to 15 years old, and quick diagnosis and treatment must be undertaken for the best chance of cure.

The fourth main category of disease is **degenerative** disease. Such diseases are far more commonly seen in older people, but children are occasionally affected by this type of condition. Examples include degenerative brain disorders such as the mucopolysaccharide diseases—for example, Hunter and Hurler syndromes—and other conditions with a biochemical basis. Many of these diseases have a genetic basis, and they must always be considered as possible causes if a toddler or school-age child loses skills that had already been learned.

Finally, **allergies** are a common cause of illness in childhood. Examples of this type of disorder are the trio of asthma, eczema, and hay-fever—so often seen in one form or another in members of the same family. In this group can also be placed certain types of food allergy, such as the allergy to the protein in wheat that afflicts children (and adults) with celiac disease. Allergy to cow's milk (often a temporary phase only) as well as other food allergies are also an important aspect of childhood illness.

(**Accidents** of all kinds, from accidental poisoning to road traffic accidents, are another important cause of distress and "dis-ease" in children. Their cause, prevention, and treatment are subjects on their own.)

TYPES OF DISEASE

Types of disease affecting children, as already suggested, can be quite different from those seen in adults and specific to the childhood years. For example, there are no adult diseases comparable to the osteochondrites, such as Perthes disease, in which certain bones become weakened and friable, causing pain, and the child loses the use of the affected body part. Specific tumors—such as Wilms' tumor and retinoblastoma—are other examples of conditions found only in childhood.

Certain pitfalls in diagnosis are caused by the ways in which children react to disease. For instance, an adult with tonsillitis will be only too well aware that his or her throat is sore and that that pain is the basic reason why she or he is feeling unwell. A child with a similar condition, by contrast, can easily throw parents off the scent by complaining of abdominal pain, making no mention at all of throat pain, even though the region can be a fiery red and very obviously infected. Such confusion may arise because the child has not developed, as yet, the verbal skills to pinpoint pain accurately, or it may be that different physiological patterns occur in childhood. Whatever the reason, knowledge of these factors will enable the true diagnosis (and hence appropriate treatment) to be made more rapidly.

Children also react to disease, such as an infection, more rapidly than do adults. All childcare givers are aware that children can wake up feeling perfectly well and bubbling over with life and energy only to become feverish, in pain, and, on occasions, severely ill by lunchtime. Fortunately, the reverse also holds true. Children can bounce back to health in a surprisingly short time.

STAGE OF DEVELOPMENT

The stage of development reached when a child suffers a specific disease is also important when the long-term effects of illness are being considered. For example, a severe infection of one kind or another contracted during the early stages of speech development can cause marked delay in the acquisition of this skill. However, if a similar infection is acquired at a much later date, when speech and language are fully developed, the illness will have little or no effect on the child's verbal skills.

Similarly, a child's other developmental milestones—for example, walking and the finer motor skills, such as hand dexterity—can be affected more seriously by an illness during the critical months of development of the particular skill.

All in all, disease in children can be a minefield of diagnostic pitfalls, but it can be very satisfying and rewarding when the correct detection of clues leads to appropriate treatment and the cure of a childhood illness! On the other hand, heartache can regretfully occur when a disease is found to be, at the present state of knowledge, incurable. In such cases, the child's life can at least be made as comfortable and fulfilling as possible when care givers have accurate knowledge of the natural history and course of the condition.

Acne

INCIDENCE

The exact incidence of acne is not documented, but the condition is so common in adolescence as to be an almost normal part of growing-up. Fortunate indeed are the adolescents who escape with no signs of acne at all. Boys are more commonly affected than girls.

While adolescence is by far the most usual time of life for acne to occur, newborn babies occasionally have the typical lesions, usually on the cheeks. No treatment is necessary at this early age, as the acne will disappear spontaneously by the time the baby is around 6 weeks old.

Acne can also make its first appearance at around 3 months of age, again most often on the cheeks only. At that age, acne can be more of a persistent problem, and it will need treatment if it is to clear within the next two years. In these cases, there is often a strong family history of acne, and these children frequently have a return of the typical rash later in life, most commonly in the adolescent years.

HISTORY

Acne has been described in the literature from time immemorial. The word *acne* comes from the Greek word *acme*, meaning the pinnacle, or prime, of life—an apt description of adolescence, physically at least!

CAUSATION

The rash of acne arises from the sebaceous glands. The most common areas of the body to be affected are the face, back and chest. The sebaceous glands secrete a substance known as sebum. This substance largely consists of fatty chemicals that perform the vital function of lubricating the skin. With the appearance of acne, a number of changes take place in these glands:

- there is an increase in the amount of sebum produced;
- there is an increase in the fatty acid content of the sebum;
- the lining of the ducts becomes thickened to produce the typical comedones (or "blackheads") of acne (the blackening is due to an increase in pigment, not to dirt!);

5

■ a specific bacteria causes inflammation to occur around the glands.

These changes, occurring in varying degrees in different people, give rise to the typical rash of acne.

There are a number of underlying factors that, in turn, cause these changes to take place.

At puberty, there is an increase in the male **hormones,** especially in boys. Girls also have some male hormones in their bodies, and at puberty girls can experience a temporary imbalance in the proportions of male and female hormones.

In girls, **fluid retention** can be a premenstrual problem, and it is thought to have a bearing on the increased incidence of acne during premenstrual days.

These two factors are the most important causes of acne, the temporary hormonal imbalance being the most important factor.

Other factors include the following:

Certain aspects of **diet** have been said to affect the severity of the lesions in some boys and girls. Chocolate, coffee, and nuts have all been implicated, but the relevant types of food are an individual variation.

Some specific **oils** used in certain industries—and even the oil used in some cosmetics—can lead to a more extreme rash. DDT and some herbicides have also been implicated in the onset of acne.

Drugs, including steroids, some anticonvulsant drugs, and some of the combined types of oral contraceptives, can be triggering causes.

The **time of year** appears to have a bearing on the severity of the rash: summer light has a good effect on the condition, and acne is often at its worst during the winter months.

CHARACTERISTICS

There are two main types of acne described—in addition to the type seen in young children.

Acne vulgaris is by far the most common type. Around 40% of boys between the ages of 17 and 19 years old have some degree of this type of acne. Girls seem to suffer from acne at a slightly earlier age (around 16 to 18), a time that probably coincides with the maximal time of hormonal imbalance.

The skin of individuals suffering from acne often tends to be more oily than normal because of the increased production of sebum. In severe cases, the rash can leave scars that remain visible throughout life, serving as a permanent reminder of a person's youth.

Acne conglobata is a severe form of acne in which the pimples are so numerous that they become confluent, with many inflamed and cystic nodules filled with pus. In extreme cases, there can be associated fever and general feelings of ill-health. This condition is especially common in the tropics.

MANAGEMENT

Management of acne can require long-term sensitive handling during the adolescent years, when it is important—for both boys and girls—to look as good as possible. Young people should be reassured that their pimples will eventually clear, and there are a number of treatments that can be tried in the meantime.

It is important to keep the skin as **clean** as possible to reduce the incidence of infection of the pimples with the bacteria specific to acne. Holding a hot damp cloth to the face, or bending over a bowl of steaming water, will open up the pores. If this treatment is followed by gentle washing with unscented soap, infection will be reduced to a minimum. Such cleansing should be done two or three times a day.

There are a number of over-the-counter **topical preparations** for the control of acne on the market. Most of these ointments act by dissolving the plug of dried skin cells in the pimples (or comedones) as well as by reducing the oiliness of the skin. **Vitamin A,** manufactured as a cream, can also be helpful.

Sunlight has a beneficial effect on acne. Ultraviolet light is a less effective treatment than natural sunlight, but it is useful in the winter months when natural sunlight is at a minimum.

Tetracycline or **erythromycin** in tablet form is also helpful in some severe cases of acne. It is often necessary to take this form of medication on a long-term basis because several months can pass before any improvement is seen. (Tetracycline interferes with the action of some forms of contraceptive pills and must not be given in pregnancy. Therefore, this form of treatment may not be appropriate for some adolescent girls.)

Other medications are available to treat extremely severe cases of acne. These must be given with care, and must be very carefully monitored because serious side effects can occur.

A number of ways of controlling the condition may have to be tried before a treatment that suits the individual person with acne is found. Reassurance that the rash will eventually disappear is an all-important ingredient in the treatment. It must be stressed that any treatment must be continued on a long-term basis.

PREVENTION

There is no known means of prevention for acne, apart from being born into a family that has no history of acne! Scrupulous cleanliness of the affected areas and persistence with treatment are the best ways of controlling the condition.

THE FUTURE

Acne in adulthood is rare, although it is thought that around 1% of men and 5% of women have some degree of acne in middle life.

Anorexia Nervosa

Eating disorder.

INCIDENCE

Anorexia nervosa is most commonly found in adolescent girls, but the condition is by no means unknown in younger children. Also, in a recent survey, it was found that one quarter of the cases in this younger age group were boys.

In the younger age group (8–14 years old), the condition can reach a dangerous state without being recognized—probably because anorexia nervosa is generally considered to be solely a disease of older girls.

The incidence of this condition appears to be on the increase in Western nations.

CAUSATION

In adolescent girls, psychological factors are probably the prime instigators in the onset of anorexia nervosa. Today's representatives of fashion all shout the message that "thin is beautiful," and the fashion-conscious teenager will respond to such influences. Individuals with anorexia have a distorted image of their own body shape—insisting that they are fat, ugly, and overweight, when, in fact, their bones stand out starkly and unattractively.

At a deeper level, fear of adulthood with all its responsibilities and stresses can subconsciously lead the adolescent to seek ways of keeping a childish anatomy and physiology. The menarche—typically occurring when a girl is around 12 to 14 years old—is a definitive sign of approaching maturity, and anorexia commonly begins around that time.

Overly close, intrusive family relationships, particularly between mother and daughter, may also have a possible bearing on the etiology of anorexia nervosa.

Children with this condition tend to be perfectionists who worry about many aspects of everyday living.

CHARACTERISTICS

The onset of anorexia nervosa is usually insidious, the young person using all kinds of tactics so that parents will be unaware of how little she or he is eating. Food is hidden; small helpings are frequently requested; meals are avoided; strange diets are tried; and the individual may induce vomiting and/or use excessive doses of laxatives, particularly in the later stages of the disease.

The physical features of this disease are very nonspecific, but anorexia nervosa should be suspected when several of the following behavioral and physical characteristics combine.

Behavioral characteristics

Moodiness, with depressed thoughts and comments, is common among anorexic children.

Such children will also demonstrate a **loss of interest** in most aspects of living, including activities previously much enjoyed.

There is often a marked interest in some aspects of **food,** including such emotional issues as animal rights and hunger in the world.

Clinical depression may be associated with the other manifestations of anorexia nervosa.

Physical characteristics

Weight loss is, of course, the most important sign. When children are in their years of active growth, lack of normal weight gain can also be significant. The ratio of weight and height appropriate for the child's age must be taken into consideration.

Obvious lack of appetite is another possible characteristic of anorexia. Most children 8 years old and older have healthy appetites, unless they are suffering from an intercurrent infection or some other disorder. (A transient anorexia often follows such events, but appetite usually picks up again quickly.) After a long day at school or pursuing some activity, a healthy child generally consumes the evening meal with relish, while children with anorexia will make all kinds of excuses for avoiding this meal.

The child may complain of **abdominal pain or discomfort,** and she or he may use such symptoms as an excuse for not eating.

Complaints of **tiredness and dizziness** may also be features of this condition.

Upon examination, the following features can be seen in the anorexic child, in addition to thinness and a poor weight (in relation to age and height):

- **cold hands and feet** due to poor circulation;
- **dry skin;**
- **low blood pressure;**
- a **slow pulse,** and, later on in the disease, **slow, deep breathing.**
  (In the late stages of the disease, the child's breath will have the characteristic odor of acetone (an odor reminiscent of pears). The odor is due to the breakdown of body tissue as a result of virtual starvation.)

Bulimia nervosa is an allied condition, which can coexist with anorexia nervosa. Persons with bulimia will "binge," or overeat, and then induce vomiting or consume excessive purgatives in an effort to counteract the effects of overeating.

Ultimately, if the anorexic child refuses fluids as well as food, **dehydration** can occur. Signs of this serious condition are sunken eyes, a weak pulse, low blood pressure, and a decreased output of urine. The child is then gravely ill and in urgent need of treatment. Death can occur—and does in some 5% of cases of children with severe anorexia nervosa. Death can be due to hypothermia, to an infection that the weakened body is unable to counteract, or to irreversible changes in body chemistry.

MANAGEMENT

Treatment for severe anorexia nervosa is difficult and long term. A period of hospitalization—preferably in a specialized unit—is often needed. The initial aim is to **hydrate** and **feed** the child until a normal pattern of eating has been re-established. Recovery obviously cannot happen overnight—the child who has eaten practically nothing will need to increase food intake at a slow, but steady, rate. The help of a dietitian is valuable in ensuring a balanced diet.

In very severe cases, where the child is adamant that she or he will not eat, nasogastric feeding may need to be undertaken as a last resort during the initial stages of treatment. (Occasionally, the suggestion that this procedure might be done is sufficient to start the child eating again.)

Once the initial physical hurdles have been overcome, it is necessary to tackle the basic cause of the original onset of the anorexia. A child psychiatrist with a special interest in anorexic children can guide the liaison that must take place among doctors, social workers, dietitians, and others concerned with helping the child and the family.

Treatment for any underlying depression must also be undertaken; antidepressant drugs may be prescribed.

THE FUTURE

A **recurrence of anorexia nervosa** can be triggered by stress (examinations, boy/girl relationships, etc.), and new episodes must be quickly contained with the help of specialists.

Final adult height may be adversely affected, if anorexia occurs during a crucial stage of growth, particularly during a growth spurt.

Fertility may be affected in women who had anorexia. Fertility problems are due to damage to the ovaries and uterus during the time of poor nutrition. The incidence of this effect is not fully known.

Osteoporosis is also thought to be a possible late effect of anorexia nervosa. The early teenage years are a crucial time for the development of a healthy skeleton. If virtual starvation occurs at that time, bone density may be poor when the individual is older. This effect is not fully understood.

Anorexia nervosa can be a difficult condition, first to diagnose and second to treat. Best results are obtained with early help before body changes become too pronounced or severe.

SELF-HELP GROUP

American Anorexia Bulimia Association, Inc.
165 West 46th Street, Suite 1108
New York, NY 10036
212-575-6200
http://www.aabainc.org

Appendicitis

INCIDENCE

Appendicitis is no more common in childhood than in adult life. A recent national survey in the UK found that around 3 or 4 children in every 1,000 suffer annually from appendicitis. The condition can occur at any age, but it is more usually found in persons over the age of 5 years. Appendicitis is an emergency at any age, and especially so in children. The appendix is a small, finger-like projection from the cecum, a part of the large intestine situated in the right lower part of the abdomen. In childhood, the wall of this vestigial organ is thin, and it can therefore rupture can occur more readily than in adulthood. Rupture leads to **peritonitis,** a serious condition in which the abdominal cavity becomes inflamed and infected as a result of the contents of the bowel spilling into that body cavity. Unless the appendix is removed surgically, the condition can be fatal.

CAUSATION

In plant-eating animals, the appendix fulfills a digestive function. In humans, this organ is merely a vestigial remnant, fulfilling no useful purpose at all. Inflammation caused by specific bacteria in the appendix occurs in this part of the intestine when either a kink develops in the appendix itself or when something obstructs the lumen. The offending obstruction can be anything from, for example, an apple seed to a toothbrush bristle! More frequently, however, hardened food material is found to be the probable cause of the obstruction.

Initially the inflammation is localized in the appendix, but surrounding lymph glands and other abdominal tissues quickly become involved. It is this reaction that gives rise to the typical pain of appendicitis.

CHARACTERISTICS

The correct diagnosis of acute abdominal pain in children is notoriously difficult. Appendicitis can be just one of the many causes of this common childhood symptom. Much experience is necessary to unravel all the clues. But it is vital that an acute inflammation of the appendix is not missed. In fact, it is preferable that a normal appendix is removed than an inflamed—and potentially dangerous—one is missed.

Typically, the signs of appendicitis are:

- A sudden onset (over an hour or so) of **colicky abdominal pain.** This pain can be continuous or, alternatively, come in spasms. The pain usually starts around the area of the umbilicus. In adults, the pain typically moves, after a short time, to the right lower part of the abdomen. This movement can also occur in children, but frequently the child describes the main pain as remaining in the center of the abdomen. If the appendix is in an unusual position behind the main bowel, the pain is felt more in the loin region.
- Most children with appendicitis have at least one episode of **vomiting.**
- **Diarrhea** is also a relatively common feature in the early stages of childhood appendicitis. It is then followed by constipation.
- There is commonly, but not invariably, a **rise in temperature.**
- The child will prefer to **lie still,** in a fetal position, in an attempt to reduce the pain.

INVESTIGATIONS

There are no specific investigations that need to be made to confirm the diagnosis of appendicitis, although **ultrasound or a CT scan** may be used as an aid to diagnosis. It is, however, wise to **test the child's urine** to exclude a urinary infection as the cause of the pain.

MANAGEMENT

The treatment for appendicitis is an operation to remove the appendix. Even if the appendix is found not to be inflamed during the operation, it is removed to prevent trouble at any later date. A short stay in the hospital is necessary following surgery. If the child has been seriously ill prior to operation, intravenous fluids may be necessary for a short time during and after the operation. Dissolvable stitches are used, so their removal does not pose a risk to the child.

Early **movement** is encouraged, and the child is allowed to play. Children are very good at judging the limits of their abilities under such circumstances.

A normal **diet** can be given as soon as the child asks for food.

Schooling can usually be resumed two or three weeks after an appendectomy. The timing of the child's return to school will depend, of course, on how ill the child has been prior to surgery. No restrictions need to be put on activities, but any complaints of pain after physical activities should always be fully investigated and quieter pursuits advised for a short time.

COMPLICATIONS

There are few complications to a straightforward appendectomy, but **infection** can occasionally occur locally around the incision. Such infection is readily cured with antibiotics.

THE FUTURE

There are no long-term problems following appendicitis. Indeed, if the appendix has been removed, appendicitis need never again be considered as a possible cause of future abdominal pain!

Arthritis

ALTERNATIVE NAMES

Juvenile chronic arthritis (the name most commonly used); juvenile rheumatoid arthritis; Still disease. (The two latter names are rarely used.)

INCIDENCE

There are no exact figures available for the incidence of juvenile chronic arthritis, but it is probably the most common of the connective disorders seen in childhood. It is seen in all countries and is thought probably to have an incidence similar to that of diabetes in childhood: around 2 children in every 1,000. While arthritis is therefore not a particularly common disease, affected children will need much monitoring and care.

The usual age of onset is younger than 5 years old, but the condition can occur at any age throughout childhood. Boys and girls are equally affected.

This form of rheumatic arthritis must not be confused with acute rheumatic fever, which was a far more common, and serious, disease of childhood until the middle of the twentieth century. Acute rheumatic fever is also primarily a disease of connective tissue, and it can have arthritis as part of its symptomatology. There is a strong association between acute rheumatic fever and infection with a particular type of streptococcal bacterium, which is not the case with juvenile chronic arthritis. The incidence of rheumatic fever has declined as a result of three factors: better living conditions, which diminish infection rates; the advent of penicillin, which is active against streptococci; and a decline in the virulence of the specific *Streptococcus* bacteria.

HISTORY

Dr. George Frederic Still first described the condition (or group of conditions) now known as juvenile chronic arthritis in 1896. Until fairly recently, the condition was referred to as Still disease. Since the specific subtypes have been classified more stringently, the disease has been renamed juvenile chronic arthritis.

CAUSATION

Juvenile chronic arthritis is part of the wide group of diseases that affect the connective tissues of the body. Several factors are thought to be involved in the causation of the disease: first, there is probably some genetic predisposition to this group of diseases; second, an autoimmune process (in which the body starts attacking its own tissues) may be involved; and, finally, added infection may play a part in the onset.

CHARACTERISTICS

Arthritis and rheumatism are wide-ranging disorders of connective tissue, there being more than 200 different types known. Several of these can affect children. Three of the more common modes of onset, and subsequent progress, of the disease will be described.

Systemic juvenile chronic arthritis

This type of arthritis begins with a feverish illness. The **fever** occurs daily and can be as high as 105° Fahrenheit. This fever usually resolves at some time during the day, only to return again within the next 24 hours. This intermittent pattern can make the diagnosis difficult to differentiate from a number of other diseases that have an intermittent fever as part of their initial symptomatology.

At this early stage, the attendant signs and symptoms associated with fever occur— **a rapid pulse, shivery feelings, lack of appetite,** and **irritability. Glands** in the neck, armpit, and groin become swollen and tender. A **rash,** of a typical coppery-red color, also affects some children during the initial stages of the illness. This rash is especially noticeable following a hot bath, but it is not irritating.

At this early stage, **arthritis** with tender swollen joints may be completely absent, only to appear a few weeks, or even months, later. (This fact can, of course, make for great difficulties in diagnosis.)

Investigations for systemic onset disease

While there are no specific tests for juvenile chronic arthritis, **blood tests** will show abnormalities. The **white blood cell** count is high; **anemia** is usually present; and the **erythrocyte sedimentation** rate, or C-reactive protein level, is raised. (These are nonspecific tests that are positive in any condition where there is any degree of inflammation, due to any cause.

All these findings can be due to any number of other conditions, and they are therefore of no specific help in diagnosis, but, of course, all give added clues.

To add to diagnostic difficulties, a positive rheumatoid factor, found in the blood in other types of onset of this disease, is rarely found when the disease has this acute systemic onset.

Polyarticular juvenile chronic arthritis

This type is easier to diagnose in early stages than systemic onset disease for a variety of reasons.

A number of **joints** will be **painful, red,** and **swollen.** The joints involved in this process are usually the smaller ones of the body—wrists, finger joints, ankles, and, at times, knees. The specialized joints in the neck (those with limited movement) can also be involved. As a result, the child may complain of neck pain and may hold his or her head over to one side. The temporomandibular joint (concerned with opening the jaw) is also often involved. For this type of juvenile chronic arthritis to be diagnosed, five or more joints should be involved in the disease process.

A **low-grade fever** can be present, but it is quite unlike the variable, spiking fever pattern associated with the acute systemic onset of the condition.

Swelling of the **lymph glands** may occur, but not to such a marked extent as with the onset of the systemic type.

Investigations for polyarticular type

A **blood test** specific for the rheumatoid factor can be done, but it can be somewhat unhelpful—some, but by no means all, children will have a positive rheumatoid factor. It is important, however, that this test is done, as those children who have a positive reading do not have as good an outlook for the future as those children whose tests are negative.

Pauciarticular juvenile chronic arthritis

This type of arthritis is diagnosed when four, or fewer, joints are involved in the disease process. More than half of the children with juvenile chronic arthritis fall into this group. Symptoms include:

- **pain, redness,** and **swelling** of one to four joints of the body; the knees and ankles are most frequently affected in this subgroup of arthritis;

- children with this type of juvenile arthritis have **none of the generalized effects** seen in the other two subgroups; they remain generally well, with no fever, throughout the course of the illness.

MANAGEMENT

Adequate **rest** is an important factor in the treatment of children with juvenile chronic arthritis. Complete bed rest is only necessary for those children seriously ill with the disease—namely, those children with the serious systemic type or with many painfully affected joints. However, all children with the condition will benefit from an adequate night's rest—around 12 hours every night is a good working figure; even if the child does not actually sleep, nighttime bed rest is valuable and an hour or two of rest in the middle of the day is advisable.

Physical therapy plays an important part in the treatment of juvenile arthritis. Once the most acutely painful stage of joint involvement is over, an exercise program tailored to the individual needs of the child should be planned. The aim is twofold: first, to maintain the mobility of the joints; second, to keep up the strength of the muscles around the joints.

Hydrotherapy pools are valuable for these treatments. The warm water makes painful joints easier to move, and the buoyancy afforded by the water makes exercise less stressful for muscles. The aim is to put all joints of the body through a full range of movement every day.

Splinting of joints is also an important part of treatment. During the acutely painful stages of the disease, specially fitted splints should be worn at night to prevent deformity occurring. The splints will have the added benefit of preventing pain caused when joints are inadvertently moved during sleep. During the day, splints can give relief from pain when worn over joints in constant use—such as, for example, wrists during a school day.

The **drug treatment** of juvenile arthritis is complex and depends upon the type and severity of the disease in each individual child. **Aspirin,** or one of the many other nonsteroidal drugs, is the first medicine to be tried. When drugs are prescribed, each individual child will need careful monitoring to assess both the benefits from the drug and unwanted side effects.

Second-line drugs include **gold** and **penicillamine** preparations. Again, these must be careful prescribed and monitored by doctors specializing in the treatment of juvenile arthritis.

Finally, **steroid** drugs are used if treatment with the other groups of drugs fails to control the disease. The decision to use steroids over the long term is one that must not be taken lightly, because of the serious side effects that can result from prolonged use of these drugs. In children, retardation of growth, as a side effect, is an ever-present worry. Mixtures of all these drugs, tailored to each child's specific needs, can be used.

Local steroid injections into specific joints can give short-term relief and prevent total loss of function in the joints in selected cases.

Schooling can be continued once the acute stage of the disease is over. Limitations on physical activities will need to be sorted out between the educational staff and health professionals. Generally speaking, competitive sports such as football, hockey, and sprinting are not suitable. Even if the child feels able to compete, energies should be tactfully diverted into other activities more suitable for potentially damaged joints. For example, competitive swimming is one sport in which the child with juvenile arthritis should be able to keep up with peers. Also, as a leisure activity, cycling is suitable. (It is advisable to determine that the atlantoaxial joint—at the base of the skull—is stable before commencing any sport.)

For children with severe arthritis, **special schooling** may be necessary.

Occupational therapists can provide valuable help for the severely affected child who has difficulty with such everyday activities as dressing, going to the bathroom, or eating. Therapists can also suggest suitable activities when long periods of bed rest become necessary for children severely affected by the disease.

COMPLICATIONS

In addition to joint problems, a condition known as iridocyclitis can affect the **eyes.** Long-term inflammation of different parts of the eye can lead to cataract formation and/or glaucoma. These later effects are seen more frequently in children who have the pauciarticular type of juvenile chronic arthritis. Surgical treatment for cataracts may be necessary at a later date, and glaucoma may need surgical or drug treatment.

Complications can also arise from **long-term drug treatment,** especially if the steroid drugs have to be used for any length of time. **Growth retardation** can occur under these circumstances, together with an increased susceptibility to **infections** of all kinds. **Osteoporosis** (thinning of the bones) can be a consequence of the long-term use of steroids—or of the disease itself.

THE FUTURE

Juvenile chronic arthritis is a long-term disease, and the future will depend on both the type of disease and the response to treatment. Some children will be severely handicapped throughout life by their arthritis. As they grow older, they may need surgery to replace disorganized and useless, painful joints or to release tight muscles that are causing deformity. However, 70 to 80% of sufferers will lead useful, independent lives.

In less severe manifestations of arthritis, adequate splinting during exacerbations of the disease will do much to keep deformity to a minimum. Physical therapy, practiced on a long-term basis, is vital to preserve mobility of joints and muscle strength.

SELF-HELP GROUP

American Juvenile Arthritis Organization
c/o Arthritis Foundation
1330 West Peachtree Street
Atlanta, GA 30309
404-872-7100
http://www.arthritis.org

Asthma

INCIDENCE

It is difficult to quote the exact incidence of asthma, partly because of problems with the precise definition of this condition. The line between "wheezy" bronchitis and asthma has been blurred, making for difficulties in quantifying incidence of asthma.

The severity of asthma varies greatly, ranging from the child with infrequent attacks and no need to stay away from school to the child who needs to carry an inhaler at all times. The latter child may also need to be hospitalized frequently to deal with severe life-threatening attacks.

Boys are affected twice as frequently as girls by this condition. There is also often a strong family history of allergies of one kind or another. It is thought that around half the children suffering from severe asthma are related to someone who has asthma, eczema, hay fever, or some other specific allergy.

Asthma seems to be less troublesome during the winter months than during other parts of the year. It has been found that the number of individuals hospitalized with asthma is highest between May and June and between September and November. These times of the year, of course, are the times when natural allergic substances are most prevalent.

Asthma is known worldwide—only in the rural areas of developing countries is the disease rare. The highest rates of increase are seen in developed nations. This fact suggests that environmental factors have a strong influence on the incidence of asthma.

HISTORY

William Osler, the well-known Canadian physician who was a professor of medicine at Johns Hopkins during the nineteenth century, considered asthma to be a "neurotic disorder." Half a century later, this view had undergone a marked change, with asthma being recognized as a distinct clinical entity and treatment for attacks being routinely prescribed. In the late 1960s, Dr. Roger Altounyan, a physician deeply interested in immunology, discovered the action of the drugs that today are used to prevent asthma attacks.

CAUSATION

Hereditary factors, as mentioned previously, play a part as to whether a child suffers from asthma. Any child whose parents or siblings have one of the atopic allergic problems is more likely to be asthmatic than a child who has no such family history. ("Atopy" can be described as any allergic condition in which specific antibodies are produced in response to a variety of outside stimuli. Such conditions include hay fever, eczema, allergic rhinitis, and allergic conjunctivitis.)

The **environmental factors** that can be involved in the onset of an attack of asthma are legion. They are usually specific to each sufferer, although frequently more than one substance, or group of substances, can initiate an attack.

Probably one of the most common allergens (those substances to which a child reacts) is the common **dust mite.** Dust mites are minute creatures that inhabit houses—especially beds—of even the cleanest and most hygienic of beings. Mites probably account for the large number of nighttime attacks of asthma.

Dogs, cats, horses, and other **creatures with fur** trigger asthma attacks for many children. This sensitivity effectively precludes beneficial contact with domestic pets and other animals.

Feathers in pillows can cause attacks of wheezing in susceptible children.

Secondhand smoke is also a potent factor in the onset of an asthmatic attack.

External factors such as **pollen** from trees and flowers in springtime can be the triggering factor for many children. Media reports of high pollen counts can alert asthma sufferers to take extra precautionary measures.

Air pollutants from the exhaust fumes of cars and trucks have recently been postulated as a possible cause for the increase in asthma, particularly in cities. It is thought that this form of air pollution does not in itself cause asthma, but it increases the allergic response in susceptible people, including children. Microscopic particles from diesel oil have also been implicated, but this finding has yet to be clarified.

Viral infections of the upper respiratory tract are also implicated in the onset of an attack of asthma. (Infections due to bacteria are not thought to produce such a response.) This causative factor is thought to be of special importance in children, who seem very prone to infection of this kind.

Intolerance to certain **foods** has been considered a factor. This hypothesis is difficult to prove conclusively either way, although some parents are quite certain that some foods—specific to each individual child—will bring on an attack of asthma.

Exercise, particularly in cold air, will tend to exacerbate asthma in some children. If the outside temperature is warm and humid, an attack of asthma is not so likely to occur.

Psychological factors can be a causative trigger for some children. Excitement or worry can result in an attack. Even laughter can precipitate a short-lived wheezy attack, as can crying.

CHARACTERISTICS

In children, a diagnosis of asthma should be considered if:

- **wheezy breathing** is heard under specific, but isolated, conditions (e.g., during the course of a viral respiratory infection; during exercise, especially outside on a cold winter's day; or at times when the pollen count is high); which conditions cause the attack will depend on the individual susceptibility of each child;
- the child has a **cough,** especially during the night;
- the nighttime cough is associated with **breathlessness.**

On **physical examination,** there is often little to be learned from listening to the child's chest, particularly if the exam is done between attacks of wheeziness. The main purpose in performing this form of examination is to exclude other reasons for the wheezy attacks, which will give specific findings.

A **diary** kept by the child's parents, showing when asthmatic attacks occur in relationship to exercise or exposure to any of the other well-known trigger factors, is of great value—both in helping to make the diagnosis and in planning treatment.

In severe, long-standing cases of asthma there can be **poor growth** and **chest deformity.**

Diagnosis of asthma can be quite difficult because relatively few features occur in this common, and potentially serious, condition. It is of interest to note what exactly is happening in the bronchi of the child with asthma:

- a narrowing of the bronchi by the action of the specific allergen on the tiny muscles in the walls of these structures;
- swelling of the mucosal lining of the bronchi;
- sticky secretions partially blocking the narrowed lumen of the bronchi.

When all these three abnormalities occur together, it is no wonder that the child has difficulty in breathing! The "breathing out" part of the cycle is especially affected during an asthmatic attack.

INVESTIGATIONS

A **chest X-ray** is taken initially. The X-ray will not show any changes specific to asthma, but it will exclude any other reasons for the child's attacks of wheeziness—such as, for example, something stuck in one of the bronchi. (It is amazing how long a peanut can remain stuck in a small child's bronchi with only wheezy breathing to announce its presence.)

Readings from a **peak flow meter** are the most helpful investigation. These readings can vary at different times of the day, and also in relationship to physical activities.

Skin tests for allergic substances are of limited value. A child with any allergic symptoms will probably react to most of the common allergens, such as dust from mites, pollen, or animal fur.

MANAGEMENT

Management is a specialized subject, and in some parts of the country, there are clinics devoted entirely to the management of asthma. Treatment will vary depending on both the frequency and severity of the attacks of asthma.

All parents of children with asthma should endeavor to identify, and remove as far as possible, the **triggering factors** in the household. For example, the **household pet** may have to be found another home if contact with the susceptible child brings on asthma. Measures to reduce the amount of **house dust** are important. "Damp dusting" can help, as can vacuuming of mattresses in an attempt to get rid of dust mites. Synthetic fillings for pillows and cushions should be tried in case the child is allergic to feathers. (As an emergency measure for getting rid of the mite, try popping the pillows and blankets into the freezer for a while. The dust mite detests the cold!)

Smoking should be strongly discouraged if any family member has asthma. This rule should also apply to visitors to the house.

Sporting activities should not be discouraged. It is better to give the child suitable medication so that she or he can take part in the school activities than to stop her/him from taking part. (It can be difficult to maintain a balance between avoiding overprotection of the asthmatic child and allowing him/her to run the risk of a severe asthmatic attack.

Parents should receive full **explanations** of their child's disease, along with advice on how to handle everyday activities and events.)

Schooling for asthmatic children should be along as normal lines as possible. Teachers should be aware of the child's respiratory problems and should know what action to take if an asthmatic attack should occur during the school day. Many children will need to take their inhalers— containing the medication that has been prescribed for them individually—to school. Easy and quick access to these inhalers is important for children who are too young to manage their medication for themselves.

Psychological factors, such as anxiety and over-excitement, should be reduced to a minimum. (Parents should be aware, however, that youngsters sometimes learn that they can get their own way by working themselves up to initiate an attack of asthma.)

If there is thought to be any possible **food intolerance,** the potentially offending foods should be avoided.

DRUG TREATMENT

There are three main groups of drugs used in the treatment of asthma.

Bronchodilator drugs act by relaxing the muscles around the bronchi. It is the constriction of these muscles that causes the bronchi to narrow in response to an allergen in an attack of asthma. The most commonly used drugs in this group are the ones that act on specific muscle receptors, which are known as **beta agonists.** They can either be taken by mouth, used in an inhaler, or used in a nebulizer. The way in which these drugs are taken will depend on the age of the child and the severity of the asthma. They are only available on prescription. (There are other types of bronchodilator drug available, but these can cause problems with side effects and so are rarely prescribed. Strangely enough, some of these drugs are available for sale in pharmacies without a prescription. It is very unwise to buy and give these nonprescription drugs to children. *Always* contact your doctor if your child has a wheezy cough.)

Corticosteroid drugs act mainly by their potent anti-inflammatory action, which reduces both the swelling and mucous secretions in the bronchi that are a result of the allergic reaction. These drugs can be taken either orally or by an inhaler. Side effects can occur with corticosteroid drugs when taken by mouth if they are used on a long-term basis. One of the most important of these side effects is the suppression of growth, which must be controlled. Serious side effects do not occur when these drugs are taken by inhaler, although infection with "thrush" (a fungal infection) can occur in the child's mouth if the inhaler is used over any length of time.

Nonsteroid drugs are also used to prevent attacks of asthma. (These were the important drugs discovered by Dr. Altounyan in the 1960s.) Sodium cromoglycate is the most frequently used drug in this group, and it has revolutionized the treatment for asthma. It is used in inhalers on a regular basis—usually four times a day—to prevent asthma. It can also be used immediately before undertaking any activity known to precipitate an attack—for example, horseback riding.

The drug treatment of asthma is a complicated one, needing constant review over the years. It is especially necessary to monitor drugs for asthmatic children, as the severity and pattern of their asthma can vary throughout the years of growth. Special asthma clinics are the ideal way to monitor the various possible drug regimens.

The treatment of an acute, **life-threatening attack** of asthma is very specialized. First aid measures include rapidly giving a specifically prescribed medicine, providing adequate fresh air, putting the child in the most comfortable position (usually sitting forward and leaning on a table), and calling emergency services.

Parents should be warned not to overemphasize their child's asthma.

THE FUTURE

For about half the children with asthma, it is a condition that will burn itself out in childhood, so that very few, if any, attacks are suffered in adulthood. It is impossible to predict which child will continue to suffer from asthma throughout life, but a strong family history of allergic disease may indicate a life-long condition.

SELF-HELP GROUP

Asthma and Allergy Foundation of America
1233 Twentieth Street, N.W., Suite 402
Washington, DC 20036
202-466-7643
http://www.aafa.org
email: info@aafa.org

Birthmarks

The term *birthmark* probably should no longer be used, as it implies that these marks happen at the time of birth. In reality, these skin marks are due to some abnormality in the structure of the skin or the underlying blood vessels. However, it will take many years before the term *birthmark* disappears!

INCIDENCE

The incidence of birthmarks is dependent on the type under discussion. The incidence of some types is not precisely known, and only a subjective impression is possible. The majority of children, however, have delicate skin with few marks to mar the surface. When birthmarks do occur, they are immediately recognizable, when other internal problems will go unnoticed.

It is worth remembering the multitude of functions performed by the skin when considering any abnormalities of this vital structure. It is often not realized how many important aspects of body maintenance and health are controlled by the skin. It:

- covers and protects all the underlying tissues from external injury, excess ultraviolet light, bacteria and fungi in the immediate environment, and excess fluid loss;
- assists in the regulation of body temperature, by means of the sweat glands situated in its structure;
- acts as a sensory organ of touch;
- acts as a synthesizer of vitamin D from sunlight;
- serves as a good indicator of health or disease. (Just think of the number of conditions—especially in childhood—that have a rash as part of the disease process.)

Birthmarks usually affect only a relatively small part of the skin; skin function is ordinarily not affected, but the cosmetic appearance of a mark, particularly on a baby's skin, can give rise to much concern.

The following are the most common types of birthmark.

Stork Bites (also known as salmon patches)

Stork bites are small reddened areas, visible from birth, which are seen most commonly on the back of the neck and on the eyelids. (The position of the marks on the back of the neck give rise to the name—the myth being that the baby was carried in the beak of the stork in this position, so leaving the mark!) There is no treatment required for such marks, which will usually fade within the first year of life, although the marks on the back of the neck can persist for longer.

Nevi

The term *nevi* refers to a large group of skin blemishes, which can be subdivided into two main groups—those that are black or brown in color and those that tend to have a reddish coloration and arise as a result of an abnormality in the blood vessels.

Congenital melanocytic nevi (CMN)

This rather complex name means that the nevus is present from birth (congenital) and arises from the pigment cells (the melanocytes) in the skin.

Incidence: It is thought that around 1.5% of the population have one or more of these nevi somewhere on their body.

Causation: It is possible that this condition is inherited in a dominant fashion; therefore, it is worthwhile to inquire if any other member of the family has similar skin markings.

Characteristics: These nevi are present at birth and can be tiny or large—they can exceed 20 centimeters in diameter. Their appearance can be **lobulated** with an irregular edge, and some can become **hairy**. The black or dark-brown color makes them very noticeable on persons with light complexions.

Complications: There is debate about whether or not there is a significant risk of these nevi becoming **cancerous** in later life. Such cancer rarely occurs during the childhood years, and it is more likely to happen to the larger nevi. Any rapid change in size or any redness around the edge of the blemish should alert parents to obtain medical advice.

Management: The way these skin markings are managed is very dependent on their size and the position on the body. Small nevi can easily be removed if they are in a very noticeable area. Larger nevi are more difficult to remove successfully and skin grafting may be necessary. Surgeons with expertise in dealing with these lesions will be needed to give advice on the relative benefits and risks of removal.

Laser treatment can remove the superficial pigmented cells and improve the skin's appearance but will not completely cure the problem.

The future: This type of nevus tends not to grow bigger of itself (unless the rare malignant changes occur, of course). Such nevi do, however, enlarge in proportion to the growth of the child.

Vascular nevi

Vascular nevi are lesions based on an underlying abnormality in the blood vessels. There are two main types:

1. Hemangiomas (also known as strawberry nevi)

Characteristics: Strawberry nevi are not usually present at birth, but they make their appearance during the first few weeks of life. The nevus begins as a whitened area—often on the face—that grows rapidly to become a lobulated, bright-red swelling. This rapid growth can continue for as long as six months, by which time the size can be worryingly large and obvious.

In the natural sequence of events, the size of the lesion—after the period of rapid growth has passed—remains constant for a varying length of time. Then, grayish areas appear over the surface and the lesion begins to steadily shrink in size. In 90% of cases, the nevus will disappear completely by the time the child is 9 years old.

If the nevus is on the baby's face and is growing rapidly, the mark can cause parents much understandable distress. It seems impossible that this bright red swelling, which so mars their baby's appearance, will ever disappear on its own. It can be helpful to have available "before and after" photographs of babies with similar nevi to show parents that the appearance of the skin really can improve.

Complications: during the period of rapid growth, ulceration of the surface of the nevus can occasionally occur. The nevus can then become infected, and antibiotics are necessary to prevent later scarring. If the nevus is near the baby's mouth or nose, feeding and/or breathing can be difficult. Under these circumstances, expert advice is needed as to how best to deal with the problem.

Management: With a relatively small strawberry nevus that is not in a difficult position, nothing needs to be done except to reassure the parents that this blemish will eventually disappear. Routine **measurements** of the size of the lesion, together with assessment of the size of the graying areas, can help boost morale during the months and years in which the nevus is shrinking. For the very large or rapidly growing marks—or those nevi that have become ulcerated—**steroids** will help to slow the growth, while antibiotics may be prescribed to control any infection. When the nevus has reduced in size, there may be some loose tissue remaining, which may require **plastic surgery** to obtain a smooth outcome. Laser treatment can also be a useful adjunct in difficult lesions.

2. Port-wine stains

Port-wine stain is the very descriptive name given to a group of nevi that are due to a malformation of the capillaries—the tiny blood vessels linking arteries and veins all over the body.

Incidence: It is thought that about 1 in every 10,000 babies is born with this type of nevus. Both sexes can be affected.

Causation: There may be a genetic factor involved, but this supposition is not certain.

Characteristics: Port-wine stains are present at birth and can occur anywhere on the body, although, unfortunately, it is often the face that is involved. Usually only one side of the face is affected. Unlike strawberry nevi, port-wine stains are flat and do not disappear spontaneously. They start off as small, pinkish spots of varying size, which coalesce to form what appears to be a sheet of colored skin. This color changes over time and becomes a purplish hue.

Complications: Again unlike strawberry nevi, ulceration does not happen in a port-wine stain, although later in life the lesion can become much more raised and lobulated. In a very small number of babies, a port-wine stain can be indicative of problems with the blood vessels in other parts of the body. Sturge–Weber syndrome is the most serious example of such a condition.

Management: A number of treatments have been tried over the years. These include surgery followed by skin grafting, various forms of radiotherapy, carbon dioxide ice, and cosmetic coverage. The best results seem to be obtained by the use of lasers. This treatment needs to be done in short bursts over a period of time.

The future: Except in the few cases of babies who have a serious and widespread abnormality of blood vessels, a port-wine stain will only have cosmetic consequences in later life. The cosmetic problems should not be trivialized, however, especially if the lesion is an obvious one on the face. Good cosmetic cover for marks on the face and psychological acceptance are mainstays of living with a port-wine stain. Hopefully, treatment with lasers will become more successful and widespread.

SELF-HELP GROUP

Vascular Birthmarks Foundation
P.O. Box 106
Latham, NY 12110
877-VBF-LOOK (weekdays) or 877-VBF-4646 (evenings and weekends)
http://www.birthmark.org
email: Linda@birthmark.org

Bronchiolitis

INCIDENCE

Bronchiolitis is the most common lower respiratory tract infection in babies under the age of 1 year. The peak age at which this particular infection occurs is 3 months, and most episodes of infection occur during the winter months.

The infection can be severe, and around 2% of all babies with this disease will need hospital treatment. Babies who already have other types of heart or lung disease, such as, for example, a congenital heart problem or cystic fibrosis, will be the most severely ill with the infection. Babies living in homes where smoking is common are prone to more attacks of bronchiolitis. Similarly, a family history of asthma, as well as over-crowded living conditions and poverty, predispose infants to recurrent attacks of bronchiolitis. Some authorities suggest that babies who subsequently develop asthma, or another allergic condition such as hay fever or eczema, are the ones most likely to suffer severely from this infection.

Boys seem to be more likely to be affected than girls. This finding is possibly explained by the fact that boys have marginally smaller air passages than girls.

HISTORY

Figures show that deaths from bronchiolitis have been steadily decreasing over the past two decades, but this infectious condition can still be source of worry.

CAUSATION

The most common causative organism in bronchiolitis is the **respiratory syncytial virus (RSV).** This virus causes much misery to the population at large, and it is thought that around 50% of all babies will have been infected by the time they are 1 year old. There are a number of different strains, and an episode of illness due to one strain will not provide immunity against other strains. Therefore, repeated infections, with similar symptoms, can occur.

RSV is an especially infectious virus and is passed on readily by droplet infection from the respiratory tract or by hand contact. Therefore, it is important that good hygiene is practiced when taking care of a baby with bronchiolitis to avoid passing on the infection to other children.

Other viruses can also cause bronchiolitis, but they are less commonly implicated than RSV.

CHARACTERISTICS

Bronchiolitis is an inflammation of the tiny air passages leading to the alveoli of the lungs where the actual gaseous exchange of carbon dioxide and oxygen takes place.

The illness starts in a similar way to a head cold, with a **runny nose** and a **fever.** A **cough** develops within two or three days and the baby will **wheeze** as each rapid breath is taken. Breathing will become more rapid, and the area of the body below the ribs will be sucked in with each breath.

As the infection worsens, **feeding difficulties** can be experienced. These are due to the problems the baby has in coordinating swallowing with the rapid difficult breathing. On listening to the chest, **crackles and squeaks** can be heard throughout the lungs.

As the disease progresses, the baby can become exhausted by the effort of breathing. **Cyanosis**—a blue coloration of the skin due to lack of oxygen—can also occur in severe cases.

MANAGEMENT

Babies with a mild attack of bronchiolitis can be safely tended at home, but hospital treatment will be necessary if the baby becomes:

- **toxic,** with a rise in temperature and breathing rate;
- **exhausted** by the effort of breathing;
- **difficult to feed;**
- **cyanotic.**

Medical advice is necessary in all but the mildest of infections. Decisions about possibility of subsequent hospitalization need to take into account home circumstances as well as the severity of the infection.

In the hospital, the baby's general state will need to be continually monitored and adequate fluids and nutrition must be provided. In severe cases, **assisted ventilation** of the lungs will be required. The baby should be disturbed as little as possible during this time.

Antibiotics play no part in the treatment of this viral infection. It is only if secondary infection with bacteria occurs—as seen by the worsening of the baby's condition with a rise in temperature and obviously infected nasal discharge—that antibiotics have any effect on the course of the illness.

An antiviral drug has been tried in the United States, but it has been found to be of the greatest use for babies who have bronchiolitis on top of an already severe lung problem, such as cystic fibrosis.

PREVENTION

While there is little that can be done to completely exclude infection with bronchiolitis, the following can reduce the incidence:

- the household in which the baby lives should be a **nonsmoking** one;
- **good hygiene practices,** such as hand washing and control of coughing and sneezing, should be observed;
- particular care must be provided for infants with other **underlying heart or respiratory conditions;**
- early medical involvement should be sought for young babies having **feeding difficulties** due to breathing problems.

For many years, attempts have been made to produce a **vaccine** against RSV; so far there has been no permanent success, but further preparations are currently being tested.

THE FUTURE

Babies who have had an attack of bronchiolitis often have recurrent "wheezy" episodes throughout early childhood. A few will subsequently develop asthma.

Bronchitis

INCIDENCE

Bronchitis is a common condition, especially during the cold winter months. Much confusion has arisen—and still arises—over the distinction between "wheezy bronchitis" and asthma. (This issue is discussed further in the entry on asthma.) Bronchitis is an inflammation of the bronchi—the cartilaginous tubes leading from the trachea (windpipe) to the alveoli of the actual lung tissue. It is in the minute alveoli that the actual gaseous exchanges take place, and when infection reaches that part of the lung, it is known as pneumonia.

While children up to the age of 5 years old suffer, on average, from around six upper respiratory tract infections every year, relatively few children develop bronchitis.

Folklore suggests a link between teething and bronchitis. In reality, there is no connection between this infection and the entirely normal process of cutting teeth, although it is possible that the pain and upset that some children suffer when their teeth are erupting can lower their resistance to infections, including bronchitis.

The incidence of bronchitis in older children is variable, a mild attack of bronchitis sometimes occurring with an upper respiratory infection. Those children who have recurrent episodes of "wheezy" bronchitis probably suffer from asthma.

CAUSATION

Bronchitis usually arises from a viral infection. These infections typically begin in the nose and throat, and then descend, in some children more frequently than others, to the lower respiratory tract. It is less usual for there to be a bacterial cause for bronchitis, although a bacterial infection may follow an initial viral infection.

Measles and whooping cough—a viral and a bacterial infection, respectively—are always complicated by bronchitis to some degree.

CHARACTERISTICS

Bronchitis usually follows, or is seen in conjunction with, an **upper respiratory tract infection.** The symptoms of the latter are well known to everyone: a runny nose, a sore throat, and possible a mild fever.

The one diagnostic symptom of bronchitis is a **cough.** This cough is dry in the early stages, but within a day or two, it will become loose, and **yellowish sputum** may be coughed up. Children, however, tend not to cough up secretions but to swallow them. This practice can on occasions cause **vomiting.**

A **wheeze** can also be heard in some children with bronchitis. In bronchitis, the wheeze is caused by air passing through bronchial passages that have been narrowed by infection. As mentioned previously, this symptom can also be a manifestation of asthma.

The child may or may not have a mild **fever,** together with general feelings of **malaise.** The child may also be reluctant to eat.

On listening to the child's chest with a stethoscope, the typical sounds of the air passing through the inflamed bronchi can be heard.

MANAGEMENT

In a straightforward case of bronchitis, antibiotics are of no value, as the infection is usually viral in origin. (Antibiotics have no efficacy against viruses.)

A **light diet,** with plenty of **fluids,** and play in a warm room is all the treatment that is necessary.

If the cough becomes an excessive irritant, keeping the child (and the rest of the family) awake at night, **cough syrup** can be given. A mixture containing an expectorant and mucolytic is preferable. Medications that have a cough suppressant are not advisable because the cough is part of the body's natural defense mechanism, helping to remove infected material from the lower respiratory tract.

If the child with bronchitis is particularly wheezy, medication to dilate the bronchi can be prescribed to good effect.

Attendance at school should cease until the worst of the cough has cleared and the child is feeling able to cope with the physical demands of school again.

In an uncomplicated attack of bronchitis, the cough will clear within a week to ten days, and the child will return to full health.

COMPLICATIONS

Secondary bacterial infection of the bronchi can occur. Under these circumstances, the cough will show no signs of improvement, and may even grow worse. The child may also become more feverish, or run a fever where there was none before. Antibiotics will be needed to clear the infection under these conditions.

Pneumonia, where the infection reaches the alveoli of the lung, can be a complication of bronchitis. This infection can be due to either a virus or a bacterium. (Pneumonia can occur, of course, without a preceding upper respiratory tract infection or bronchitis, especially in premature babies, children who have some congenital defect, or those children who are malnourished.)

The infection can affect either the whole of a lung (or both lungs) or a segment or lobe of a lung. The former is known as bronchopneumonia and the latter as segmental or lobar pneumonia.

The child with pneumonia will be seriously ill. There will be a rapid rate of respiration—this finding is in direct contrast to the picture seen with bronchitis, where the respiratory rate is within normal limits. The child's nostrils will be dilated as she or he struggles to get air into the lungs. The cough will be persistent and irritating, and fever will be high—altogether a far more severe set of symptoms than is seen with an attack of bronchitis.

Investigations if pneumonia is suspected include a chest X-ray, a throat swab, and a blood test to be examined in the laboratory for the infecting organism.

Hospital admission is necessary for the child severely ill with pneumonia. An oxygen tent and intravenous fluids may be necessary during the initial acute stages. Antibiotics are necessary to cure the infection. Even if the initial pneumonia was caused by a virus, secondary infection with bacteria is common.

Older children with a less severe attack of pneumonia can be tended at home, if the home circumstances are suitable. Parents should always be encouraged to contact their doctor again if they are at all worried about their child's condition.

THE FUTURE

Uncomplicated bronchitis will have no permanent after-effects on the child. It is when the symptoms become blurred with those of asthma that long-term effects—due to the asthma—may occur.

Celiac Disease

INCIDENCE

Celiac disease appears to be predominantly a condition seen among people of European origin. While it is not unknown in the Far East and Africa, the incidence in those areas does not appear to be as high as it is in North America and Europe. This finding may, however, be due to differences in the ways in which disease types are recorded.

HISTORY

This condition was recognized in children more than 100 years ago, but it was not until the early 1950s that the relationship between celiac disease and the eating of wheat-flour products was noticed by Dr. Dicke. Later in the 1950s, the pathological changes in the small intestine were described.

CAUSATION

Celiac disease is one of the many malabsorption conditions found in both adults and children. There are a great number of conditions—some mild, some serious, some temporary, some permanent—in which the malabsorption of food is the basic cause.

In celiac disease in particular, there is an allergic response of the small intestine to gluten, a substance found in wheat and wheat products. Some sufferers are also allergic to a similar substance found in barley, oats, and their products.

It is thought that a basic immunological fault in the individual with celiac disease causes the pathological changes seen in the small intestine following the consumption of gluten-containing products. There appears to be a higher than normal incidence in some families, although no specific genetic link has, as yet, been found.

CHARACTERISTICS

The age at which an affected child will show signs of celiac disease varies between 9 and 18 months. The onset follows fairly soon after the beginning of mixed feeding, when wheat products are first introduced to the diet.

There are two main ways in which celiac disease manifests itself. On the one hand, there can be a relatively acute onset with **diarrhea, lack of appetite,** and a marked **abdominal distention.** Over the succeeding weeks, there is a loss of weight. In the child with fully developed, untreated celiac disease, the contrast of the grossly distended tummy with the starkly thin buttocks and thighs is very marked.

A slower, more insidious onset may occur, marked by signs of a **lack of growth** both in height and weight and the development of an **iron-deficiency anemia.** (The importance of serial measurements of height and weight, recorded on a percentile chart, is highlighted once more in this condition.)

The child with celiac disease will tend to be miserable, complain of stomach aches, and generally be unwell.

INVESTIGATIONS

In addition to the clinical and serial measurement signs noted, examination under the microscope of a small piece of the intestine is necessary to confirm the diagnosis. This test is known as a **jejunal biopsy.** (The term refers to the specific part of the intestine, the jejunum, that is examined.) In this procedure, the child swallows a tiny instrument, known as the Crosby capsule, which removes a small part of the intestine. The capsule is then recovered from a bowel movement.

On examination under the microscope, the appearance of the lining of the small intestine is quite unique if celiac disease is present. The normal picture is of a series of "ridges" in the membrane, which make for a large surface area through which absorption of food materials can occur. In persons with celiac disease, the ridges (in adults these structures are more finger-like and are known as "villi") are completely absent, and as a result, very little food can be absorbed.

Specific **blood tests** for iron and for a specific antibody against gliadin (the protein in the gluten) can help with the diagnosis, as can a measurement of the **fat excreted** in the bowel movements. These tests are nonspecific, however, and they can also be positive if the child has certain other diseases of the small intestine. Therefore, it is always advisable to perform a jejunal biopsy before treatment is started. Ideally, another jejunal biopsy should be done after several months on a gluten-free diet, when the microscopic picture of the small intestine will appear normal.

MANAGEMENT

The treatment for celiac disease is a **gluten-free diet,** and within a few weeks, a vast improvement will be seen in the young sufferer. She or he will begin to gain weight; diarrhea (if it has been a problem) will cease; and she or he will have more energy and be altogether a happier, easier-to-manage child.

At first sight, the exclusion of all wheat-containing foods from the diet can seem daunting, but with advice from a dietitian, parents and childcare givers will soon become used to the new regimen. According to present knowledge, a gluten-free diet should be followed for life.

It is vital that the child with celiac disease should have **regular check-ups** to ensure that normal growth and development are maintained. At these check-ups, any problems with diet can also be resolved.

Some authorities advise a **gluten challenge** after two or three years on the gluten-free diet. Wheat-containing foods are reintroduced into the diet, and another jejunal biopsy is performed. If the appearance of the intestinal sample under the microscope regresses to that seen before the gluten-free diet, the diagnosis of celiac disease is 100% correct. These serial jejunal biopsies may reveal, however, that the gluten intolerance was a transient phenomenon, rather than a permanent condition.

Children for whom the diagnosis was delayed may need **dietary supplements** of vitamins and minerals for a short time until those important substances can be properly absorbed again. The absorption of iron and vitamins D and K can be especially affected.

COMPLICATIONS

Complications are unusual, and if they do occur, they are readily rectified.

An **iron-deficiency anemia** can occur in children when the diagnosis is delayed or difficult. Oral or injected supplements of iron will readily cure the anemia.

Rickets caused by the malabsorption of vitamin D can also occur very occasionally if the diagnosis is delayed. Here again, supplements will halt this process.

During the difficult period of **adolescence,** strict adherence to the gluten-free diet may be less than perfect! No adolescent wishes to eat different foods from their contemporaries, and individuals that age often rebel against advice. Only minimal effects are initially seen, but there will eventually be a return of the malabsorption symptoms. Sensitive handling during this period can reduce problems to a minimum. (This problem may not strictly qualify as a "complication," but it is nevertheless a situation that frequently occurs and one to be remembered during the adolescent years.)

THE FUTURE

There has been a reported increase in the incidence of intestinal cancer in people with celiac disease, but this hypothesis has not been fully elucidated. Also, it is not entirely clear whether strict adherence to a gluten-free diet throughout life has any bearing on this future possibility.

SELF-HELP GROUP

Celiac Disease Foundation (CDF)
13251 Ventura, Blvd., Suite 3
Studio City, CA 91604-1838
818-990-2354

Chicken Pox

ALTERNATIVE NAME

Varicella.

INCIDENCE

The exact incidence of attacks of chicken pox in children is not known. It is, however, a common and highly infectious disease occurring most usually in children between the ages of 2 and 8 years old. Chicken pox is found all over the world, except in a few isolated communities. In children, the disease is usually a mild one with few complications or permanent after-effects. In adults contracting the disease, the picture can be different, serious illness occasionally being the result. From this point of view, it is preferable that chicken pox should be contracted during childhood rather than adulthood. (Introduction of the infection to isolated communities who do not generally suffer from chicken pox can also result in serious health problems.)

There are two groups of children for whom the risk of serious consequences of chicken pox is quite great: children who are receiving immunosuppressant drugs for some other condition and very young babies. For both these groups, chicken pox can be a life-threatening disease, which can necessitate hospital admission.

CAUSATION

Chicken pox is caused by a virus. Immunity gained by a naturally acquired attack of the disease is usually lifelong, so that second attacks are extremely rare. It is not unusual, however, for an attack of shingles to occur in later life, often following a period of general debility. Shingles is caused by a reawakening of the virus, which has lain dormant in the body for many years. On the other side of the coin, a child can contract chicken pox from an adult with shingles.

Chicken pox has an incubation period of 14 to 21 days with, most usually, the next member of the family showing signs of the infection on around the 16th day. The infection is most likely to be transmitted during the first few days of symptoms, when the virus is present in the saliva.

43

Droplet infection from the breath or during sneezing or coughing is the common mode of passage of the virus.

CHARACTERISTICS

The infection starts, in many children, as a mild, nonspecific illness with a general feeling of **malaise** and frequently a **low-grade fever, headache,** and occasionally a **sore throat.** (In other words, the illness is initially very similar to the symptoms and signs of a common cold.) It is not until the appearance of the typical rash that chicken pox can be said to be the cause of the original symptoms.

The **rash** passes through three stages. First, there is a raised, red, discrete rash, which, within a very short time, will become blistered. It is at this stage that the diagnosis of chicken pox will become obvious. Second, after two or three days, the clear fluid within the vesicle (or "blister-like" spot) will become cloudy and assume a yellowish color. Third, as the disease progresses, these spots will crust over, leaving a scab that, if scratched off, can leave a permanent white scar.

The rash appears in crops, with two or three days between the appearance of each crop. Because of this "cropping," all of the various stages of the rash can be seen at the same time.

The distribution of the rash of chicken pox is also very specific. Initially, the rash is confined to the chest and face, with covered areas of the body having more spots than exposed parts. By the third day, the rash spreads to the limbs. In mild cases, relatively few spots occur, but in severe cases, the rash can be very extensive and even include the palms of the hands and the soles of the feet. In all but the very mildest of attacks, the rash is also found on the mucous membranes of the mouth and ears, and, in the most severe cases, in the eyes and the vagina.

Severe **irritation** is one of the most unpleasant aspects of chicken pox. This symptom makes its appearance soon after the vesicles have started to crust over. Scratching at this time can cause **scarring** to occur or, more seriously, **infection** of the spots with bacteria.

INVESTIGATIONS

As a general rule, an uncomplicated attack of chicken pox does not require specific investigations. The diagnosis is made on clinical grounds alone.

The virus can be isolated in the laboratory from the fluid in the vesicles during the first three or four days of the rash. This test is usually an unnecessary exercise, except in unusual cases where there is some doubt about the diagnosis.

MANAGEMENT

General sympathetic care is all that is needed for a mild, uncomplicated attack of chicken pox. A **light diet** with plenty of cool drinks is sensible during the early stages when the child feels generally unwell and has a fever. Confinement to bed is unnecessary—quiet play in a warm room is all that is needed.

 Calamine lotion and frequent **tepid baths** will do much to allay the irritation of chicken pox. If itchiness is a problem in spite of such treatments, an **antihistamine cream** can be tried. Fingernails should be cut as short as possible to prevent injury through scratching. **Aspirin must never be given to children with chicken pox** because of the link between the use of this analgesic in cases of chicken pox and the development of Reye syndrome.

 Schooling can be resumed one week after the onset of the rash if (and only if) the child is feeling perfectly well. Once the spots have crusted over, transmission of infection is no longer a problem—the scabs contain no active virus. Many children are unnecessarily sent home from school because they still have a few crusted spots. It is only if the child is still feeling unwell that she or he should be at home.

COMPLICATIONS

Complications are rare with an attack of chicken pox.

 Secondary infection of the rash, due to scratching, is the most usual complication of this mainly mild disease of childhood. Antibiotics may be necessary if the infection is severe.

 Pneumonia can occur in adults or in children with autoimmune disorders. Children who do not have another underlying disease will not suffer from this complication.

 Encephalitis is another possible, but rare, complication.

PREVENTION

A chicken pox vaccine has come into widespread use and is generally given along with other childhood vaccinations. The vaccine either prevents or greatly decreases the symptoms of chicken pox in children who receive it.

Quarantine measures are unlikely to succeed as chicken pox is such a highly infectious disorder at a time before the diagnosis becomes obvious.

THE FUTURE

There are generally no future problems following an attack of chicken pox. The only possibility is an attack of shingles later in life due to the reactivation of the dormant virus.

Congenital Dislocation of the Hip

INCIDENCE

In northern Europe, the incidence of congenital dislocation of the hip (CDH) is around 1 in every 1,000 births. A number of other babies—perhaps as many as 1% of all births—have "unstable" hips (i.e., hips that are potentially capable of becoming dislocated). Babies in the latter group need careful monitoring until they are walking satisfactorily.

The incidence of CDH is especially high in Japan and also among peoples who tightly "swaddle" their babies, such as Lapps and Native Americans. The hips of babies who are tightly wrapped, or "swaddled," remain in an extended, or straight, position for many hours. Thus, if there is any underlying instability of the hip, dislocation can occur more readily—and the instability may persist into later childhood.

Girls are affected five times more often than boys. Both hips can be affected or only one. In the latter case, it is more usual for the left hip to be affected.

HISTORY

Routine screening of all newborn babies for dislocated hips only began in the 1950s, and there is still much to be learned about the incidence and causes of this condition as well any long-term effects in later life.

CAUSATION

Both genetic and environmental factors can be contributory causes to congenital dislocation of the hip. These different factors will be specific to each individual child.

Direct inheritance seems to play a small part in the causation, although a definite form of dominant inheritance has been reported from one large family who had several members with the problem. It is probable that—as with many other conditions—there can be a familial tendency to abnormalities in the hip joint.

The markedly higher incidence seen in girls may have something to do with the influence of female hormones on the laxity of the ligaments surrounding joints in general and, in this case, the hip joint in particular.

Prenatal factors, such as the fetus lying in the breech position for some time, are further potential risk factors. For some obscure reason, first-born babies are more prone to CDH.

CHARACTERISTICS

The hip is a "ball-and-socket" joint in which the "ball" of the head of the thigh bone fits neatly into the "socket" on the pelvic bone.

In the newborn baby, a congenitally dislocated hip will not be noticed unless specific screening tests are done to detect the condition. It is only when the child begins to walk that the problem becomes obvious. At this time, there will be a **limp**, a very specific **waddling gait**, possible **pain in the hip,** and a **reluctance to walk far.** All these signs and symptoms are not necessarily present in each individual child, but any combination of them should alert parents to seek further investigation. Hopefully, this situation will never arise if the following tests for congenitally dislocated hips are done in the early days of life.

If only one hip is affected, it may be possible to notice in the newborn baby a **shortening** of the affected leg; similarly, at this time, a difference in the **position of the folds** in the two legs can be obvious.

There are two specific maneuvers that can detect a dislocation or potential dislocation as in an unstable hip. These tests are termed the **Barlow** and **Ortolani maneuvers.** They rely on the ability of the examiner to—very gently—test whether or not the head of the femur (the thigh bone) can be moved in and out of its normal position in the pelvic bone. (These tests do not hurt the baby or cause distress in any way.)

These screening tests need to be done three times during the first year of life—in the immediate newborn period, at 6 weeks of age, and at around 9 months of age.

It is especially important that tests for CDH are carried out on babies who are at a potentially high risk, such as:

- babies related to someone who has the condition;
- babies who were in the breech position for some weeks before birth;
- babies who have some other positional problems, such as clubfoot (an in-turning of the foot). It is thought that up to 20% of babies with CDH have some other positional difficulties.

Any question as to the stability of the hip—or hips—following these screening tests will need evaluations with ultrasound and possibly treatment with close follow-up over the succeeding weeks and months. Referral for continuing care by an orthopedic surgeon is the usual course of action.

INVESTIGATIONS

X-ray examination of the hip is unhelpful as the bones in this area of the baby's body are not as yet ossified so as to be visible on X-ray.

Ultrasound examination is of value, and research is continuing into this method of detecting CDH. At present, this method is largely used to assess babies who are found to have an unstable hip on clinical examination and babies who are at a high risk of having this problem; ultrasound is also used to monitor the success of treatment in babies with a definite dislocation or instability.

It must be emphasized that these screening procedures will not necessarily identify all children with CDH. Therefore, it is of vital importance that parents should report any worries they may have regarding their child's walking abilities—at least until the child is 2 or 3 years old, when this skill should be fully attained.

MANAGEMENT

The aim of treatment for unstable hips is to keep the head of the femur firmly in the pelvis by placing the baby's legs in a frog-like position by means of special **splints** for up to three months. This procedure ensures that as growth proceeds, stimulation to the development of the joint is correctly applied. Caring for a baby who is wearing one of these splints can cause parents some initial difficulties:

- strollers and cradles need to be wide enough to accommodate the baby lying in the "frog" position;
- diaper changing can be more difficult, as can bathing;
- rubbing of the splint on delicate skin must be carefully checked to ensure that pressure sores do not develop.

For hips that are completely dislocated, it is necessary to apply gentle **traction** until it is possible to place the hip joint into its correct position. Following this treatment, the splinting process will be necessary to maintain the position.

For dislocated hips that are late in being diagnosed, or those hips that do not respond satisfactorily to splinting, **surgery** may be necessary.

THE FUTURE

Early diagnosis and treatment typically results in a virtually normal hip joint. Where there is some residual deformity remaining in the joint, degenerative disease with possible osteoarthritis can occur later in life.

Constipation

Constipation is not a disease entity, but rather a symptom that can be associated with a wide range of conditions. Most frequently, chronic or long-term constipation is the result of an acute event (again, due to any number of possible causes) that results in temporary constipation. This symptom is included in the text because of its relatively common occurrence and because of the concern it can cause both children and their parents. Early diagnosis of the cause followed by appropriate treatment is vital for the well-being of the whole family.

INCIDENCE

Constipation is not an exciting enough condition for anyone to want to measure the exact incidence. Nevertheless, it is unusual for any day pass in which a pediatric clinic does not treat at least one child for chronic constipation.

Constipation can be defined as delay in the passage of stools, which can reach a chronic state in which the lower bowel is blocked by hard, bulky feces.

CAUSATION

Causes of constipation are multiple. There are, however, certain groups of conditions that predispose a person to this symptom.

There may be some abnormality in the intestine, such as the much narrowed segment of the intestine seen in Hirschsprung disease or some gross narrowing around the anal region.

Conditions in which the child is forced into physical inactivity can predispose her/him to chronic constipation; examples of such conditions include cerebral palsy, spina bifida, and hypothyroidism.

If the child has a high fever, she or he can become dehydrated and/or eat little food; both these facts will contribute to constipation, which, unless recognized and treated, can become a long-term problem.

The presence of an anal fissure, in which there is a tiny crack in the skin around the anus, can make defecation so painful as to put the child off going to the bathroom completely! Stools will deliberately be held back, and as a result, the feces become hard and bulky and even more painful to pass. In addition, the lower bowel will become so stretched that eventually all normal sensation of the need to defecate will be lost, creating a vicious cycle.

Unsympathetic, rigid handling of toilet training in the toddler years can result in the child becoming desperately concerned about this normal bodily function. If there are then inadequate toilet facilities at daycare or school, the problem is compounded.

It is thought that intolerance to certain foods can be a causative factor in the onset of chronic constipation. This fact has always to be considered in a child who also has eczema or asthma.

A sizable number of problems could thus be causative factors in the onset of long-term constipation.

CHARACTERISTICS

The characteristics described refer to long-term constipation and its treatment. The possible underlying causes—outlined above—will also need to be understood and treated.

The constipated child will often be brought to the doctor by parents complaining that she or he has **diarrhea!** This observation can seem paradoxical, but it can be understood when it is remembered that hard feces are blocking the lower bowel tightly, while the fluid waste-products above this blockage gradually leak, soiling the child's underwear as diarrhea might.

On examining the child's abdomen, the hardened feces can easily be felt. In a rectal examination, the solid masses can also easily be felt.

As the problem progresses, the urge to have the bowels move will diminish because of the **over-stretching of the lower bowel.** This development, of course, compounds the problem.

The child will occasionally complain of **abdominal pain** when chronically constipated. Surprisingly, however, pain is not a common complaint.

INVESTIGATIONS

It is not often necessary to do any further investigations other than the initial examination, but an X-ray of the abdomen will occasionally be used to show the extent of the constipation. (X-rays can also be useful to verify the diagnosis for the parents, who, after all, initially thought their child had diarrhea!)

MANAGEMENT

Treatment of any underlying cause for the constipation must be the long-term aim to prevent the condition recurring.

Dietary advice, preferably from a pediatric dietitian, regarding adequate fluid and fiber intake is vital.

Treatment of any **anal fissures** with a local anesthetic cream is also important. The bowel can often be effectively emptied when pain is no longer felt on defecation. To empty the bowel completely initially, it is usually necessary to give two or more **enemas.** The procedure can be done at the child's home, but it is often more satisfactory to admit the child to the hospital for a day or two so that it can be determined that the bowel is completely clear. Following this treatment, a daily dose of a **laxative** should be given to be sure that the bowels are moved at least once a day. (A stool softener such as lactulose can be used in conjunction with a stimulant such as senna.) The dosage of the laxative drugs may need to be altered until the right amount is found to produce the desired result without giving the child diarrhea. This medication will need to be continued until the bowel has been "re-educated." With the gross over-stretching of the bowel by the hard mass of feces for some considerable length of time, the child will no longer be aware of the need to visit the bathroom, but as the rectum returns to its normal diameter, normal sensation will return.

Advice on **regular**—relaxed—**times** for visiting the bathroom must be given, and followed, alongside the medical treatment. Immediately after breakfast is a good time (if an adequate period of time can be found at this often stressful time of the day). Food in the stomach can initiate the "gastrocolic" reflex, which helps with bowel elimination.

A system of **"star charts"** can sometimes be helpful (as with enuresis—see elsewhere in the text). The child is encouraged to note on the chart the days when the bowels have been successfully moved. Emphasis must always be placed on success, rather than note taken of failure.

This regimen will have to be continued for some considerable time before full success is achieved—months rather than weeks. Both parent and child can become disheartened by the need for lengthy treatment. Therefore, it is important that adequate **support** is given throughout this time by all involved—pediatricians, medical staff, and dietitians.

In the event of no—or little—success over a considerable period of time, there may be need for **further investigation** to be sure that no anatomical or other abnormality is the source of the chronic constipation.

It is also worth checking that the child has no hidden **fears** about visiting the bathroom.

THE FUTURE

The future is, of course, dependent upon the basic cause of the constipation in childhood. If there is no underlying abnormality, constipation need no longer be a problem in later life, as long as a suitable diet and regular bowel movements are made a part of everyday living.

Croup

INCIDENCE

This upper respiratory condition affects children 18 months old and older. After the child is 2 years old, attacks of croup become less common.

CAUSATION

Both bacteria and viruses can be the causative organisms involved in croup. The most usual bacteria to be involved are the *Streptococcus, Staphylococcus,* and *Hemophilus influenzae* bacteria. Most infections, however, are caused by the parainfluenza virus or respiratory syncytial virus. All these organisms are common causes of recurrent upper respiratory tract infections in children—and adults.

Some children with allergies have frequent attacks of croup. These attacks are not thought to be always necessarily associated with an infectious process but are rather a hyperactive response in the airways. Younger children are often more susceptible to this type of croup—possibly because of the relatively smaller size of their air passages.

CHARACTERISTICS

Children with an infectious type of croup will start with the usual symptoms of a head cold—a **runny nose, poor appetite,** and a **fever.** Within 24 to 48 hours, a **barking cough** follows, and with each breath drawn, there is a loud, harsh wheezing noise known as **stridor.** This symptom can be particularly severe at night.

The child will be restless, and the **ribs** can constrict with each difficult breath—an extremely worrying picture for parents. In severe cases, **cyanosis**—a bluish tinge to the skin—can occur. This latter sign is serious and shows that the child's airway is in danger of complete obstruction.

Children with recurrent attacks of croup have no head-cold symptoms before the onset of the harsh barking cough. There will be no fever, and stridor is less acute than with an infection. This type of croup is an altogether milder type, but it can, of course, progress if an additional infection intervenes.

Other conditions in which stridor is a feature must be excluded. For example, an inhaled peanut or other small object can give rise to a similar noise, and epiglottitis is a possibility in the younger age group that must not be forgotten.

MANAGEMENT

Children with an infectious type of croup will need urgent medical advice, because of the rapidity with which airway obstruction can occur. Depending on the severity, **hospitalization** in a unit with facilities available to deal with obstructed airways is often necessary. **Oxygen** can be necessary to aid gaseous exchange in the lungs, and **steroids** can be helpful in reducing symptoms. If the infecting organism is thought to be a bacterium, **antibiotics** will need to be prescribed.

For children with an allergic attack of croup, home remedies, such as staying in a room with a **steaming kettle** or a **vaporizer,** together with a **mild sedative**, can help. However, these remedies must never delay the call for medical help if the condition does not improve rapidly or worsens.

THE FUTURE

Croup usually ceases by the time school days start. Wheeziness, cough, and milder attacks of stridor can occur, of course, throughout life, due to both allergic and infectious causes—such as asthma and laryngitis, for example.

Deafness

Deafness itself is not a disease entity. It can be a symptom of many types of disorder, ranging from congenital and inherited problems to infections of all kinds and also injuries.

There are two types of deafness—**sensorineural deafness,** in which the actual nerves of hearing are involved, and **conductive deafness,** in which there is interference in the passage of the sound waves to the nerves of hearing. These two types will be dealt with separately as, although the outcome—deafness—is the same, etiology and treatment differ.

SENSORINEURAL DEAFNESS

Incidence

A sensorineural hearing loss affects around 1 in every 1,000 children. This figure includes those children who have a severe hearing loss—in the range 65–80 dB (decibels)—and those with a profound hearing loss—in the range of 85 dB and above.

Causation

There are several possible causative factors for this type of deafness.

Genetic deafness can be inherited in a number of ways, either as a dominant or a recessive characteristic or, in some circumstances, in a sex-linked manner. Certain specific syndromes also have deafness as part of the symptomatology (for example, Waardenburg syndrome, Usher syndrome, and Treacher–Collins syndrome).

Infections acquired either prenatally or after birth can cause sensorineural deafness. Infection during pregnancy with cytomegalovirus, toxoplasmosis, or (probably the best known of all) rubella can cause deafness. If any of these infections are contracted at a critical time in pregnancy, during the fetal development of the organs of hearing, congenital deafness can result. Infections contracted during childhood can also cause deafness as a complication. Examples of such infections include measles, mumps, and bacterial meningitis.

Problems during the neonatal period (the first four weeks of life), such as jaundice or oxygen deprivation, can result in sensorineural deafness.

Certain **drugs** can also be a causative factor. Streptomycin used to be a fairly frequent cause of deafness, and a few antibiotics, given long-term, must be watched for this side effect. Drugs given during pregnancy can also cause deafness—thalidomide was the best known example of this kind of cause. Quinine is also known possibly to have a similar effect.

Characteristics

It is vital that a sensorineural deafness in babies is diagnosed as soon as possible. If a severe sensorineural hearing loss from birth is not quickly treated, the child will not be able to develop "inner language" and so will never be able, in later life, to use language adequately.

It is important that any questions voiced by parents regarding their baby's hearing should be carefully investigated and followed up.

Babies at greater risk of deafness because of a strong **family history** of poor hearing must be checked carefully.

Vision should be watched throughout the child's early life in cases where the cause of the deafness is uncertain. For example, Usher syndrome, in which there are associated visual problems, can cause deafness.

Management

Once the extent of the hearing loss has been determined, a plan of continuing treatment and education will need to be formulated. For children with a bilateral loss, **hearing aids** will be necessary to make full use of any residual hearing they may have. Radio transmission aids are the most successful.

Services for the hearing-impaired can give much help and advice to minimize the child's handicap. This assistance will need to be continued for many years.

Many children can be happily integrated into **ordinary schools.** A few especially handicapped children will need special schooling and/or teaching by sign language. (The most appropriate and successful methods for teaching deaf children is hotly debated in educational circles. It would seem that an amalgam of all possible methods of communication would be the most satisfactory.)

Any **associated handicap**—such as, for example, the later visual problems seen in Usher syndrome—must be assessed and managed appropriately.

With specialized, and early, teaching, children deaf from birth can develop understandable speech. The importance of early intervention cannot be stressed too highly.

The future

Career choices must, of necessity, be severely curtailed for children with profound sensorineural hearing loss. Good career advice should be available from the early teenage years onward.

Later, when a **pregnancy** is contemplated, genetic counseling should be available for prospective parents who are sensorineurally deaf or have a family history of the condition.

CONDUCTIVE DEAFNESS

Incidence

Conductive deafness is by far the most common cause of deafness in children. It is thought to affect around one-third of all children between the ages of 2 and 5 years at one time or another. Although many children will improve within a few months, up to one-fifth of the affected individuals will have a hearing loss that persists into late childhood. Both boys and girls are affected.

Causation

The most usual cause of conductive deafness is secretory otitis media, which can occur following an acute attack of middle ear infection. In this condition, sticky fluid fills the cavity of the middle ear, which contains three tiny bones intimately concerned with the hearing process. (Secretory otitis media is frequently referred to as "glue ear" because of the glue-like nature of the fluid in the middle ear.) Because of this fluid, the ossicles in the middle ear are unable to work adequately. That restricts the movements of the tympanic membrane (the eardrum), so dulling hearing.

The reason why this fluid persists in the middle ear following an attack of acute otitis media is thought to be lack of drainage of fluid away from the middle ear. Normally, secretions are drained away from the middle ear into the back of the throat via a tiny tube—the eustachian tube. Following an infection, this tube becomes blocked either as a result of swelling of the tissues or by mucus. Young children are especially prone to this condition, partly because of the relative frequency of upper respiratory tract infections among young children and partly because of the small bore of the eustachian tube in this age group.

Characteristics

The child with a chronic secretory otitis media will often have a deafness of around 20–40 dB. This loss, however, may not be consistent, but fluctuating from week to week. The fluctuation can easily mislead parents into thinking that their child is just not paying attention during the periods when hearing is less than perfect. Even routine hearing tests may, at times, fail to pick up the hearing loss if the test is performed on a good day.

However, even this relatively mild degree of hearing loss can interfere with the **acquisition of speech** in the younger age groups. Speech is learned by imitation of sounds heard, and if some specific frequencies are missed by the child—because of the hearing loss—fully comprehensive speech is attained with difficulty.

In the older child, who has just started school, for example, **behavioral problems** or periods of "switching off" can occur. Problems such as these can result from the child's inability to hear instructions adequately—the child compensating in other ways for the failure in hearing. "Switching off" for short periods can easily be confused with petit mal seizures (see epilepsy) unless the possibility of a hearing loss is remembered and assessed.

Children with a conductive deafness can also be thought to be **slow learners** if the hearing problem is not recognized and treated appropriately.

Investigations

Clinical examination of the ears of a child suspected of being deaf as a result of secretory otitis media can show a range of abnormalities on the eardrum. The drum can be pulled inward and/or have an unusual, grayish color. There may also be dilated blood vessels coursing across the eardrum. The advice of an ear, nose, and throat surgeon will be needed in certain cases to determine further treatment.

Audiology tests, suitable to the age of the child, will give information as to the degree of the hearing loss. For children under the age of 3 years, distraction tests will be needed. After that age, most children will be able to cope with pure-tone audiometric tests.

Impedance audiometry can also be used in especially difficult cases to determine hearing loss. (This test measures the minute movements of the eardrum in response to sound by means of a special instrument held against the eardrum.)

Management

The best way to treat the secretory otitis media that causes conductive deafness is controversial. There are four main approaches to improving the child's hearing.

Antihistamine drugs, given by mouth, were previously thought to help reduce swelling around the eustachian tube, thereby improving the drainage of the middle ear. Along with this treatment, decongestant nasal drops were prescribed for the same purpose. Present-day experts suggest that this form of treatment is of little value.

An operative procedure—a **myringotomy**—can be performed. In this procedure, the eardrum is pierced (under a general anaesthetic) and the sticky fluid is withdrawn. In addition to the removal of this fluid, tiny ventilation tubes ("grommets") are inserted through the eardrum and left in position. The purpose of the tubes is to ventilate the eardrum in an effort to prevent further build-up of fluid. These tubes remain in position for around 1 year to 18 months, when, in the vast majority of cases, they fall out spontaneously.

Removal of the adenoids is also advised by some ear, nose, and throat surgeons in an attempt to ease the passage of fluid down the eustachian tube—but again, this procedure is controversial.

Recently, **hearing aids** have been prescribed for short periods in order to improve hearing. Results are promising, the children tolerating the hearing aids well. Most children who have suffered from secretory otitis media with an associated deafness have normal hearing by the time they are 7 or 8 years old. This outcome appears to be part of the natural history of the disease and is apparently unrelated to the type of treatment previously given. At this time, with this satisfactory result, hearing aids will no longer be required.

One further cause of conductive deafness is a **build-up of wax** in the external auditory meatus—the passage from the exterior down to the eardrum. The build-up can easily be seen with an auroscope and removed, either by a syringe or by making the hard wax more fluid with ear drops. Occasionally, it is necessary to soften especially hard wax with ear drops before using a syringe.

The future

There is rarely any return of the conductive deafness in later life. The usual, temporary, catarrhal deafness following a head cold will, of course, still occur, but it rarely persists for any length of time.

SELF-HELP GROUP

American Society of Deaf Children (ASDC)
848 Arden Way, Suite 210
Sacramento, CA 95825-1373
800-942-2732 or 916-482-0120
email: ASDC1@aol.com

Diabetes

ALTERNATIVE NAMES

"Sugar" diabetes; diabetes mellitus (the correct name for this condition, which distinguishes it from diabetes insipidus—a condition associated with disease of the pituitary gland).

INCIDENCE

Diabetes is known worldwide and among all races—with a higher incidence among persons of European descent. The incidence varies widely. Epidemiology of this disease has unearthed some fascinating facts. It would seem that parts of the world farthest from the equator (either north or south) have a higher incidence of diabetes than those countries nearer the equator. For example, the number of people with this disease in France is far lower than the number in Finland.

The average number of school children with diabetes is thought to be between 1 and 2 children in every 1,000. Diabetes is rare in children younger than 2 years old. Adolescence is the most usual time for the onset of diabetes, and in this age group there is a slight preponderance of boys with the condition.

There are two main types of diabetes—the **non-insulin-dependent type** and the **insulin-dependent type.** Children predominantly have the insulin-dependent type, although the other type is not completely unknown. Further discussion will relate to the insulin-dependent type in children.

HISTORY

Diabetes has been known as a disease entity since 1500 B.C.E. It was in the second century C.E. that a Turkish physician coined the name "diabetes" (meaning "a siphon"). At that time, the disease was thought to be a condition arising in the kidneys, due to the large amounts of urine passed in the acute disease. It was not until the nineteenth century that diabetes was known to be a condition caused by malfunction of the pancreas. Dietary measures were the sole treatment available at that time. In 1922, Drs. Banting and Best discovered that insulin could be used to treat diabetes successfully.

CAUSATION

Diabetes is caused when special cells found in the islets of Langerhans fail to produce insulin in adequate amounts. Insulin is a substance that is vital to the proper metabolism of sugars in the body. It is the incomplete—or inadequate—metabolism of sugars that gives rise to the symptoms of diabetes.

The precise reasons why diabetes occurs are not completely understood, but it is known that there are three distinct groups of factors that have a bearing on the onset of the disease.

Genetic: While diabetes is not a truly inherited disease, there are strong family links in the incidence, especially for the insulin-dependent type of diabetes most usually seen in children. Children with two diabetic parents run a greater risk of developing the disease than children who have either only one parent with the disease or no positive family history of the condition. A child with two diabetic parents and a brother or sister with the disease stands a 50% chance of also suffering from diabetes. Recent genetic studies have shown a strong association between the development of diabetes in childhood and a particular "marker" on chromosome 6. Factors other than genetic ones will then determine whether or not the full-blown disease occurs.

Environmental factors appear to exert some effect on the onset of diabetes. These factors only appear to affect people who already have some genetic predisposition. The most common of these factors is infection of one kind or another. A viral infection with the Coxsackie B or mumps virus seems especially likely to be a predisposing factor. Most of these types of infections occur during the autumn and winter months, and that fact probably explains the higher incidence of diabetes onset during these times of the year. Other environmental factors, such as chemical toxins and nutritional aspects, may also have a bearing on the onset of diabetes in people with a predisposition.

Immune mechanisms have received much interest in recent years as possible causative factors in the onset of diabetes. It is known that there is a strong association between insulin-dependent diabetes and autoimmune diseases of the endocrine glands, such as the thyroid and adrenal glands. Further research into this aspect has important implications for both prevention and treatment of diabetes.

Diabetes is a wide-ranging disorder with many factors to be taken into account when the causation is debated. All people with diabetes probably have a genetic predisposition (known or unknown in the family tree).

CHARACTERISTICS

Diabetes in 90% of children with the disease has an acute onset—usually with a history of various signs and symptoms of less than a month. In the remaining 10%, the same symptoms occur, but they appear in a milder form over a longer period of time.

Symptoms and signs of diabetes in a child include:

- **frequent passage of urine:** this symptom may show itself in some children as a return to bed wetting (or even daytime wetting) after a period of complete bladder control. It is therefore vital that all children with enuresis should have their urine tested for glucose;
- an **increasing thirst:** as the frequency of the passage of urine increases, so will the child's thirst increase;
- **weight loss:** this loss can occur rapidly in an acute onset of diabetes—the child losing many ounces in a week or two;
- **loss of energy,** together with lethargy and exhaustion, will soon become obvious; at this stage, the child is seriously ill;
- **irritation** around the vulval region in girls or the penis in boys can occur due to the passage of sugar-loaded urine;
- occasionally, **abdominal pain** and **vomiting** may be added symptoms; under these circumstances, diagnosis can be delayed if it is assumed that the pain and sickness are due to a gastrointestinal upset and a sample of urine is not tested for glucose; this type of onset occurs more often in younger children;
- in a severe case of diabetes, the **breath will have a distinctive sweet smell,** similar to that of acetone or pears;
- in a serious undiagnosed case, the result can be **coma** and **death** unless correct and immediate treatment is given.

INVESTIGATIONS

Urine tests for glucose is vital for the early diagnosis of diabetes. If glycosuria is found, there should be an immediate referral to a hospital. In a severe case, the urine will also show a positive result when tested for ketones, which are secreted because of the breakdown of bodily tissues. These chemicals account for the sweet smell on the breath of an undiagnosed diabetic.

Blood tests for glucose will confirm a high level of sugar in the blood. Levels of this blood sugar will need to be measured frequently during the subsequent treatment of diabetes.

MANAGEMENT

Acute onset of diabetes must be regarded as an emergency. Rapid **hospital admission** is necessary for treatment of the seriously ill child. **Intravenous fluids** and **insulin** are the basis of the very specialized treatment regimen.

A child with a slower and **less acute onset** will still need to be admitted to the hospital once the diagnosis is made in order to set up the regimen for the future treatment of the diabetes.

About one week in the hospital is usually necessary to find the correct dosage of insulin required to stabilize the diabetes. Much care needs to be taken to be sure that the parents fully understand the basic principles behind the twin methods of the control of their child's diabetes—diet and insulin.

Diet

For good control of the diabetes, the diet must be tailored to meet the needs of each individual child. The child may have difficulty in adhering to the new pattern of eating if the diet makes him/her feel unusual among his or her peers, and it is necessary to provide support and information to help the child to stick to the diet.

It is the intake of carbohydrate-containing foods that needs to be controlled in a diabetic diet. Regular measured amounts of this type of food must be eaten. Typically, the child will need a serving of carbohydrates at breakfast; as a mid-morning snack, at lunchtime, as a mid-afternoon snack, at supper, and as a snack at bedtime.

A system of "exchange" foods is worked out, each unit of "exchange" food being equal to 10 grams of carbohydrate. This system allows for a wide variety of foods to be included, ensuring that a balanced diet is eaten. The carbohydrate portion of the diet should consist of starchy, high-fiber foods rather than foods made from refined sugar. Starchy foods are absorbed more slowly than sugar and over a longer period of time, thereby giving better control of the diabetes. Such foods include whole wheat bread and cereals, legumes, green vegetables, and fruit of all kinds.

The amount of carbohydrate consumed in any one day should be—as a rough guide—100 grams for a one-year-old child plus an extra 10 grams daily for each added year of life. (For example, a ten-year-old child will need 190 grams of carbohydrate every day.)

Each individual child will need to have a daily diet created initially by a dietitian, together with a list of "exchangeable" foods. It is surprising how quickly both children and parents become adept at estimating the correct amount of foods that make up 10 grams of carbohydrates.

Adolescence is a particular time when dietary control can cause problems. Adolescents are not the most sensible of eaters at the best of times, and diabetic youngsters are no exception. Add to the problems of diabetes the stress of examinations, career choices, and relationship problems and this time of life can be fraught with difficulties with control. At this time, too, the child will be moving on from pediatric diabetic care to treatments suitable for adult diabetes. All these changes need sensitive handling.

Insulin treatment

The vast majority of diabetic children require insulin to control their disease. Control with diet alone is very rarely achievable in childhood.

Ideally, a regimen of insulin should match the output of insulin in a normal child. This match is virtually impossible to achieve, but each individual child must be balanced on the dose of insulin that matches his or her physiology as closely as possible.

Insulin usually needs to be injected twice a day, although some children may be able to manage on just one daily injection. There are available short-, intermediate- and long-acting forms of insulin, which can be "mixed and matched" to suit the child's individual needs. Dosage will need to be carefully monitored by a diabetic clinic once the child has left the hospital.

During the initial stay in the hospital, both parents and child must be fully informed about the nature of the disease and its control. The actual physical process of injecting the insulin must also be taught. Most children over the age of 8 or 9 years will eventually be able to give their own injections, but parents must always keep a watchful eye that the shots are done regularly and competently.

General management

The child's **school** must be informed of the child's diabetes. Teachers should know the action to take if a hypoglycemic attack (see below) should occur in school, and the staff must understand and implement such practices as giving the child some readily absorbed glucose before a period of strenuous activity.

Emotional support will be needed in the early days following diagnosis, especially if the child is the first member of the family to suffer from the disease. Parents must understand that diabetes is a lifelong condition for which, at present, there is no cure. They must also understand that a full, exciting life can still be led by their child if control of the diabetes is strictly maintained.

Careers for children with diabetes will need to be carefully chosen. The risk of hypoglycemic attacks in insulin-dependent diabetes is a very real one, and diabetic people are not usually accepted in the armed forces, the police, or fire departments because of this risk. Certain other forms of employment may also be difficult or impossible to pursue.

Hobbies, too, will need to be more carefully chosen for a diabetic child than for a non-diabetic child. Any activity in which hypoglycemia could put the child or his or her companions at risk should not be recommended.

Travel may present problems in the control of insulin levels. For example, time changes when traveling long distances can cause difficulties in the timing of injections. More—or less—activity on vacations can also make differences in the dosage of insulin necessary.

When the child is old enough to **learn to drive,** special consideration needs to be given to prevent hypoglycemia while operating a car. (All drivers should, of course, have a supply of sugar in the car at all times to counteract any hypoglycemia.)

COMPLICATIONS

Hypoglycemia

Hypoglycemia (low blood sugar) is an ever-present complication for anyone on regular insulin. A variety of factors (for example, too little breakfast after having an insulin injection or too much exercise combined with insufficient food) can upset the ratio of insulin to carbohydrates. Too much insulin or too little carbohydrate will mean that the blood sugar becomes too low, giving rise to certain specific symptoms:

- dizziness and faintness;
- nausea;
- headache;
- irritability;
- and eventual unconsciousness.

The younger child will be unable to verbalize exactly just how she or he is feeling, and may just say she or he feels "odd" or "funny." Parents and teachers must learn to know what is the matter under these circumstances and give appropriate treatment. Obviously, if the child has become unconscious, a 911 call will be necessary.

Treatment is quick and easy in the early stages of a hypoglycemic attack. A sweetened drink or a piece of candy will return the child to normal. If the symptoms progress too far, parents can be instructed to give an injection of glucagon, which works to raise the blood sugar in a confused or unconscious child.

Most hospitals will deliberately allow a child to become hypoglycemic while the parents are present so that the symptoms can be recognized—and addressed—quickly.

Later complications

Vision can be affected by diabetes, because of the effect the disease has on the small blood vessels of the body.

As a result of a similar effect on blood vessels, the **kidneys** can also be affected, as can other parts of the vascular system.

These latter complications are rarely seen in childhood. Nevertheless, it is important that good control of the disease is maintained throughout childhood in order to keep complications later in life to a minimum.

Special care needs to be taken to control a woman's diabetes during **pregnancy.** The baby will also need extra supervision after birth.

THE FUTURE

Diabetes is a life-long disease, and at present, it can only be controlled and not cured. Research is proceeding along a number of lines, including possible preventable environmental triggers, the newer types of insulin, and the introduction of less toxic immunosuppressant drugs that will allow pancreatic—or islet cell—transplantation.

SELF-HELP GROUP

American Diabetes Association (ADA)
1660 Duke Street
Alexandria, VA 22314
703-549-1500 or 800-232-3472
http://www.diabetes.org/custom.asp

Diaper Rash

INCIDENCE

Diaper rash is not a condition that has excited a good deal of research into the number of babies affected! Anyone who cares for babies will know that lucky is the infant who escapes diaper rash altogether.

CAUSATION

There are a number of possible causes for each particular type of diaper rash. By far the most common causes are simple "contact irritants." Other causative factors can be seborrheic dermatitis, added infection with *Candida* (yeast), and psoriasis. Each type of rash will need a different treatment—see below.

CHARACTERISTICS

Contact-irritant diaper rash is the reaction of the relatively thin skin of the baby to constant contact with urine and feces. Specific types of bacteria that are encouraged by the warm, damp atmosphere of the diaper add to the irritation. These bacteria release ammonia, which is in itself a potent irritant. (A wet diaper often has the characteristic smell of ammonia.)

The rash is **red** and spreads over the **whole of the diaper area**, with characteristics **patches of clear skin** in the folds of the groin.

If cloth diapers are used, they will need to be rinsed thoroughly after washing because remnants of **detergent** can be an irritant cause of diaper rash.

Seborrheic dermatitis is a common cause of diaper rash. This condition can be readily confused with eczema. The most usual place for seborrheic dermatitis to occur is on the scalp, where thick, yellowish crusts appear along the hair line. This condition is commonly know as "cradle-cap." Other areas affected are the creases of the body, such as behind the ears, around chubby necks, in elbow creases, and also in the groin area. In this last—diaper—area, secondary infection with *Candida* is especially common.

Secondary infection with *Candida*—a yeast infection—can occur on top of an irritant type of diaper rash. The rash then has an added discrete red area with a well-defined edge. Newborn babies can be infected with yeast during delivery if the mother herself has a vaginal infection with this fungus. Under those circumstances, the baby's mouth is most frequently affected, but the infection can readily spread to the diaper area. With a *Candida* infection, a cheese-like white substance can often be seen in the skin folds in addition to the red rash.

These three causes are by far the most common reasons for diaper rash. On rare occasions, a form of **psoriasis** can be seen in young babies in the diaper area. Characteristically, an existing mild diaper rash due to a contact irritant becomes more severe. Large, well-demarcated areas all over the diaper area often become bright red. It is usual under these circumstances for the typical lesions of psoriasis to appear elsewhere on the body.

MANAGEMENT

The mainstay of treatment of the common contact-irritant type of diaper rash is to **change diapers frequently,** which ensures that the skin is only in contact with urine and/or feces for the minimum amount of time. In this context, **disposable diapers** are preferable to cloth ones covered with plastic pants, which foster a warm, moist environment highly favorable for the introduction of secondary infection. At each diaper change, the baby's bottom needs to be **thoroughly cleaned and dried** and a **soothing cream,** such as one containing zinc oxide, should be applied.

It is also helpful to allow the baby to **lie without a diaper**—in a warm room—for as long as possible each day.

A diaper rash due to **seborrheic dermatitis** will need the addition of a mild **hydrocortisone cream.** The ointment will need also to be applied to other affected parts of the body. It is inadvisable to use this cream for extended periods of time on a number of different parts of the body. Therefore, if the diaper rash has not cleared within one week of this treatment, further advice as to the possible cause must be sought.

Added **infection with *Candida*** will need a different cream—**nystatin,** for example—to heal the rash. It is always a good idea when a yeast infection causes a diaper rash to **check in the baby's mouth** to eliminate any similar infection in that part of the body.

Psoriasis is a difficult skin condition to treat, and a number of preparations may need to be tried. Psoriasis is, fortunately, a rare cause of diaper rash, but it should be considered when a rash proves difficult to treat by the usual means.

THE FUTURE

Diaper rash is a self-limiting condition and will no longer be a problem once diapers are discarded.

Diphtheria

INCIDENCE

Diphtheria has been an almost unknown infection in Western nations for several decades. With the advent of routine immunization of all children against this infection since the late 1940s, the incidence has fallen dramatically. In the 1940s, tens of thousands of cases, including thousands of deaths, were reported, while in recent decades the number of cases of diphtheria reported each year has fallen to a handful, and deaths are now extremely rare.

The picture is different, however, in many other parts of the world. In developing countries, diphtheria still takes a tragic toll of young life in terms of both illness and death. In the 1990s, there were also reports of many thousands of cases of diphtheria in Russia and Eastern European countries. These numbers emphasize that continual vigilance is still necessary for the control of this infection.

HISTORY

In 1881, Dr. Theodor Klebs discovered the bacteria that causes diphtheria. Soon after that date, the toxin produced by the bacteria was described, and an antiserum was developed in 1884. The early twentieth century saw the advent of a preparation that could be used to actively immunize against the infection.

In 1913, Dr. Schick developed a specific skin test by which individuals immune to the effects of the bacteria could be recognized. This test is rarely used today, but, at times, it can still be of value in determining the immune state of people working in occupations in which they might come into contact with the diphtheria bacillus.

CAUSATION

Diphtheria is caused by a bacterium. There are three different strains of this bacterium, giving rise to illnesses of differing severity. The diphtheria bacillus produces a powerful toxin, which is the cause of many of the generalized symptoms of the illness. It is also this toxin that is responsible for the serious effects seen in the heart and the nervous system.

Diphtheria is spread from person to person by droplet infection, or from clothing contaminated by the organism. Although readily destroyed by heat and antiseptic preparations, the diphtheria bacterium can survive for several weeks in both milk and water. "Carriers," healthy people who harbor the organism with no ill-effects themselves, can also spread the bacterium.

The incubation period of the disease is between two and seven days.

CHARACTERISTICS

The severity of the infection depends on the strain of the infecting organism—the "gravis" strain producing the most severe symptoms. At times, the infection can be so mild as to pass undiagnosed—the symptoms being thought to be a relatively mild respiratory infection. The development of such mild cases, of course, poses problems for those seeking to prevent the spread of the disease—especially among unimmunized children.

In more severe cases the infection will begin with generalized symptoms of:

- **fever:** in diphtheria, fever does not usually reach as high a level as with a throat infection with *Streptococcus* bacteria, but it can reach 103° Fahrenheit, and it is important that the two infections are differentiated from one another;
- **headache and general malaise;**
- **sore throat:** this is not such an overwhelmingly unpleasant symptom as the sore throat found in an infection with *Streptococcus* bacteria, but nevertheless the condition is not comfortable. Later in the course of the illness, the diphtheritic **membrane** appears in some part of the throat. The membrane is grayish and adheres to the underlying tissues; its removal leaves the under-surface raw. Danger arises if the membrane spreads over the whole throat and soft palate—and possibly further down the respiratory tree into the larynx and bronchi—and effectively excludes the passage of air to the lungs.

As the disease progresses, with the production of the specific toxin, the child's general condition deteriorates. The heart muscle can become involved, giving rise to a **weak, irregular pulse. Blood pressure will fall,** and the child will be gravely ill. In addition, the nervous system can become involved. (These latter serious effects will be seen in an infection with the most serious strain of the diphtheria bacillus in a child who is not immunized against the disease.)

INVESTIGATIONS

Throat swabs—taken from beneath the membrane, if possible—will confirm (or rule out) the diagnosis of diphtheria.

MANAGEMENT

It is vital that **antitoxin** is given by injection as soon as possible, before the toxin has become fixed in the tissues. Once the toxin is fixed, the opportunity to counteract its effects is lost. When antitoxin is given on the first day of the illness, full recovery is the usual result.

Antibiotics—penicillin or erythromycin—will also be necessary to ensure that a "carrier" state does not result.

Tracheotomy may be necessary in severe cases where the diphtheritic membrane obstructs breathing.

Skilled **nursing care** in the hospital is necessary for children with a severe infection of diphtheria. (It is also important to remember that added complications in the heart and nervous system can occur some weeks after the initial symptoms of diphtheria are obvious.)

COMPLICATIONS

Heart: This vital organ can be affected by the toxin produced by the diphtheria bacillus. The heart muscle itself is weakened, and it is therefore unable to perform adequately its function of pumping the blood around the body. It is this direct effect on the heart muscle that causes the irregular heart beat, weak pulse, low blood pressure, and other symptoms of heart failure observed in a severe case of diphtheria.

Respiration can be severely affected if the membrane extends down into the larynx. In such a situation, the sufferer will have a hoarse voice and a "brassy" cough. Breathing will be extremely difficult, and the child will be restless and anxious.

Secondary infection of the respiratory tract by other organisms can occur, giving rise to **bronchopneumonia.**

The **nervous system** can also be affected by diphtheria bacteria. Weakness and/or paralysis of any muscle, or group of muscles, of the body can occur. For example, the muscles of the eye can be involved, giving rise to a lazy eye, or arms or legs can become paralyzed.

These effects occur late in the illness—often many weeks after the involvement of the throat.

PREVENTION

Diphtheria is entirely preventable by immunization, as is verified by the dramatic fall in the incidence of the disease following mass immunization.

In Western countries, immunization against diphtheria is a part of the routine babyhood immunization schedules. Vaccination is offered for all babies at 2, 3, and 4 months of age. A booster dose is given at school entry.

Children who are known to have been in close contact with a case of diphtheria should receive another injection of vaccine. Close family contacts should also be given a seven-day course of erythromycin to ensure that a "carrier" state does not result.

THE FUTURE

With early adequate treatment, there are no subsequent effects following an attack of diphtheria—once, of course, the period of time for the late manifestations of the disease has passed. If the toxin has severely damaged the heart muscle, however, late effects in this system of the body can be seen.

Eczema

ALTERNATIVE NAMES

Atopic dermatitis; infantile eczema.

INCIDENCE

There are a number of types of eczema, with a variation in classification. **Contact eczema** or **dermatitis** is an eczematous condition in which there is a definite correlation between the cause of the condition and subsequent effect. For example, eczema can occur in some people on contact with certain metals, such as nickel (which is often used in jewelry, scissors, and some cooking utensils), or with some of the chemicals used in rubber gloves.

Eczema affects around 5% of people, and the vast majority of these show signs of the condition in childhood—often before the age of 6 months. Boys and girls are equally liable to be affected.

Hay fever, asthma, and eczema are allergic conditions that frequently occur in different members of the same family. Some 70% of children with eczema have family members with one or another of these allergic manifestations.

Atopic eczema—the type of eczema that will be further discussed—is a genetically determined skin condition in which specific antibodies can be demonstrated in the blood. Often the "triggering" factor initiating the rash proves difficult, or impossible, to find.

HISTORY

Eczema has been known since antiquity. The word "eczema" is derived from the Greek word meaning "to boil out"—a good descriptive term for the red, bubbling nature of the rash of eczema.

CAUSATION

Genetic factors are certainly at work in the child with atopic eczema, and it may be possible to discover certain foods or conditions that make the rash worse. For example, some babies have an allergy, often temporary, to cow's milk, or they are allergic to some particular material found in clothing—wool often being a culprit here. These triggering factors have to be found by trial and error.

CHARACTERISTICS

The baby/child with eczema will usually have **dry skin,** which will be in evidence from the earliest days of life.

The typical **rash** of eczema—patches of reddened skin with small blistered spots—is extremely **irritating.** The baby will scratch, making the skin further inflamed and the discomfort even worse.

Eczema typically occurs on the baby's **face** and in the **knee and elbow creases.** In severe cases, much of the body can be covered with the rash.

Some children experience a worsening of their rash during **cold weather,** while other sufferers find the rash worst during **hot, humid conditions.** This variability in manifestations of the rash can make management difficult. Each child has to be treated individually.

Improvement in the rash is occasionally seen in children between the ages of 2 and 4 years old. Unfortunately, the remission of symptoms is often short-lived, and the eczema returns again during the school age years.

MANAGEMENT

Children with eczema have—and always will have—very dry skin. **Emollient creams,** applied twice every day, reduce this dryness and minimize the outbreaks of severe eczema. Even when the worst of the rash is absent, it is important to continue with creams to reduce dryness.

Soap and **bubble bath** have the effect of drying the skin even further, and so should be avoided by children with a dry skin. Bath oil should be substituted for other bath-time additives, and a minimum of—preferably unscented—soap should be used. Moisturizers should always be applied after a bath.

Wool is a particularly frequent irritant to children with atopic eczema (as well as children with contact eczema). Most eczema sufferers will react badly to even a minimum of wool in their clothing. **Acrylic** cloth can also have a deleterious effects in some cases. Cotton and cotton/polyester fabrics are the most suitable choices for clothing worn next to the skin. (It must also be remembered that carpets and other household items can contain a certain percentage of wool. Crawling babies with an eczematous tendency can suffer from the effects of such household furnishings.)

In comparatively rare circumstances, certain **foods** can cause eczema to worsen. This condition must be distinguished from the rapid allergic reaction known as urticaria, which arises when the specific food touches the child's mouth.

Avoidance of any factors that have worsened the eczema is an important part of the ongoing care of a child with eczema. Treatment of an acute relapse includes the following:

A **steroid cream,** applied only to the parts of the skin that have eczematous patches, will help alleviate all but the most resistant cases of eczema. These creams should be applied three times daily. Parents can become concerned regarding the use of steroid creams on their children's skin. They can be reassured that there is no danger of overuse as long as the treatment is not continued for an indefinite period.

In very severe cases, particularly in young babies where control of scratching is a major problem, **wet dressings** are of value. A moisturizing cream is applied all over the child's body, with a steroid cream applied to the worst of the eczematous patches. Damp cotton material is then wrapped over these creams. This treatment, which needs to be done three times daily and may require a short stay in the hospital, has the effect of moisturizing the skin, which aids the action of the steroid creams. The irritation is reduced and, being completely bandaged, the baby cannot get at the rash to scratch his or her skin.

If the eczema has become **infected** through repeated scratching, oral dosages of **antibiotics** will be needed. An antibiotic/steroid cream can also usefully be applied to the rash.

Sedation at night—when the irritation is often at its worst—with an **antihistamine** can also help to reduce the amount of excoriation of the skin.

Eczema is a miserable, long-term problem. Parents and children will need much **support** (preferably from a doctor who knows the ups-and-downs of the individual child's eczema) to cope with the inevitable relapses that occur. It is important to emphasize that acute flare-ups can be reduced to a minimum by constant adherence to methods that reduce the dryness of the child's skin and by avoiding known triggering factors.

School days can be unhappy for eczema sufferers if teachers and pupils are not informed of the recurrent and, of particular importance, the noninfectious nature of the condition. It is a sad sight when a child with eczema is left out of activities because of an exacerbation of the rash and the lack of understanding of his or her peers.

THE FUTURE

Eczema will be a constant, life-long concern for many of childhood sufferers. When the time comes to choose a career, jobs that could worsen the possibility of an acute exacerbation of the eczema should be avoided. Work with chemicals of any kind should be avoided, for example, and hairdressing, where there is much contact with soap products and various chemicals, is not a sensible choice.

SIMILAR SKIN RASHES

There are a number of other skin rashes very similar to the eczema described above that are worthy of mention, as confusion is common.

Discoid eczema: As the name implies, this is a true form of eczema, which appears in very specific round patches. In younger children, the upper arms and shoulders are the most frequently affected parts of the body. These patches can become very large, with a moist surface. They can be difficult at times to distinguish from impetigo. Steroid creams and moisturizing ointments are the best forms of treatment.

Seborrheic dermatitis: This condition is frequently confused with eczema, especially in younger children and babies. The common "cradle-cap" seen in children less than one year old is an example of seborrheic dermatitis. In this condition, the front of the child's hair is covered in a yellowish crust—even extending to the eyebrows at times—which, when gently removed, is seen to have a red, angry base. Other parts of the body, such as the armpits, round chubby necks, and the groin, can also be affected. Unlike eczema, this rash does not itch, and so secondary infection is not a problem. Treatment for cradle cap is to apply warm olive oil to the thick scales as a softening process before applying a specific cream to remove the surface skin. For other parts of the body, a weak steroid cream is the better form of treatment. An antiseborrheic shampoo can also be of value. Seborrheic dermatitis is unusual in later childhood, but it can return in later adult life.

SELF-HELP GROUP

National Eczema Association for Science and Education
1220 S.W. Morrison, Suite 433
Portland, OR 97205
503-228-4430 or 800-818-7546
http://www.eczema-assn.org
email: nease@teleport.com

Enuresis

ALTERNATIVE NAME

Bed wetting.

INCIDENCE

All young babies are wet at night as well as during the day. By the age of 3 years, many children are dry by day, and a few are also dry at night.

By the time they are 5 years old, most children have ceased wetting the bed, except, perhaps, on a few occasions (when sick with a cold or some other infection, for example). However, around 10% of children at that age are still enuretic at night on a regular basis. The figure falls to 1% or less by the time adolescence is reached.

Boys tend to take longer to achieve night-time bladder control than do girls.

CAUSATION

For convenience sake, enuresis is divided into primary and secondary enuresis. Primary enuresis is said to occur when a child has never been dry at night apart from, possibly, a few odd occasions. Secondary enuresis refers to cases when a child who was previously dry at night starts wetting again.

Primary enuresis may be due to a physical abnormality in the renal tract, or a neurological cause. It is important to exclude any such physical abnormality before commencing treatment for the enuresis. Developmental delay in this particular aspect of growing up may be the sole cause of the problem, and it is by far the most common cause of primary enuresis.

Secondary enuresis is also common. There can frequently be found a precipitating cause for the onset of bed wetting after, perhaps, many months of dry beds. The arrival of a new baby, starting school, marital disharmony, or the death of a grandparent are all examples of stressful events in the life of a child who only has precarious bladder control.

Social deprivation and low intelligence can also be possible factors in both forms of enuresis.

CHARACTERISTICS

The characteristics of enuresis are obvious: the child awakens to find urine has been passed in the bed but has no memory of urinating. It is important that parents and childcare givers understand that bed wetting is not a purposeful act on the part of the child. She or he is genuinely unaware that the bed is wet when waking initially. Therefore, punishment has absolutely no part to play in the treatment of enuresis.

Sometimes, other factors noted in the child's **behavior** are associated with enuresis. For example, difficulties at school or temper tantrums can be signs that the child is under stress.

Daytime wetting is also found in some children with nighttime enuresis. This sign can point to some abnormality in the renal tract or to a urinary infection. Both these conditions must be excluded before treatment of enuresis begins.

Enuresis also has a definite **familial pattern.** Parents of children with enuresis frequently admit to being late in achieving bladder control themselves. If that is the case, they may have a more sympathetic outlook on the problem than those parents who had no such bladder difficulties themselves when young.

INVESTIGATIONS

First, the **history** of the time of onset, duration, and any treatments already tried must be carefully ascertained.

Next, all children with enuresis should have a **clinical examination** with special reference to the urinary tract and any possible neurological problems. Included in this examination, for example, must be palpation of the abdomen to be sure that the kidneys are not enlarged. If anything abnormal is discovered, an ultrasound examination is done to confirm the clinical findings.

Testing the reflexes (for example, knee and ankle jerks) will give information on the working of the nervous system, which is closely connected with bladder control.

A **sample of urine** must be sent to the laboratory to exclude any possible infection in the urinary tract that could have a bearing on the enuretic problem. A "dip-stick" test of a sample of urine should also be done to exclude glycosuria (passing of excess sugar in the urine).

Enuresis is rarely—if ever—the sole sign of diabetes in a child, but this disease should be considered as a possible cause for the bed wetting.

MANAGEMENT

In nine out of ten cases of children who wet the bed at the age of 5 years, the problem will resolve itself within a few years without any specific treatment. However, much distress, to both parents and child, can occur along the way unless help is given. There are several paths that can be followed to speed up normal developmental progress of this particular aspect of growing up. Until around 5 years of age, it is unwise to begin any systematic treatment. A relaxed attitude by parents, without censure for wet beds, will often result in a sudden succession of dry beds. Merely talking about the problem and learning how common it is can exert a magical effect on the whole family.

If such simple measures have not succeeded, however, there are a number of ways in which help can be given.

"Star charts": by the time that parents of the enuretic child seek professional advice, this form of help—in one form or another—has often already been tried. Basically, the idea behind such charts is to encourage children to "log" for themselves successful dry nights.

Enuresis clinics, which are run by some pediatricians, will have available standard charts of various kinds. These all put emphasis on success rather than failure. In many cases this ritual, initiated by someone outside the immediate family, can be successful within a few weeks. If there is no, or little, success with this simple method after three to four months, other forms of treatment are indicated.

"Lifting" the child from sleep when parents go to bed and taking him/her to the bathroom can be tried along with the star chart. If no success is gained by this method—or if the child becomes distressed by being awakened—it should be stopped.

Alarms: The alarm is probably one of the most well-known and advertised treatments for enuresis. It consists of a detector pad, powered by a battery, on which the child lies, separated by a sheet. If urine is passed through the sheet on to this pad, the circuit is completed and the alarm sounds. There are a number of different types of alarms available. Some make a loud buzzing noise when the circuit is completed (often waking the whole household!), while others only emit a minimal sound from a device pinned to the child's nightclothes.

It is important that parents and the child should be shown together how to arrange and test the alarm, as they can become disillusioned if the alarm fails to sound when urine has been passed in the night. It is important that follow-up, by someone skilled in the use of these alarms, is done on a regular basis. Minor adjustments, or repairs to the alarm, can make all the difference between success and failure.

If there has been no success with the alarm after three or four months of use, it is advisable to cease using this method for six months or so, and then to try again. Success rates with the alarm are good—around 80%—if used properly and with a positive attitude.

Other measures include:

Regular patterns of emptying the bladder during the day should be encouraged.

Emotional stress of any kind should be discussed with parents and the child. The causes of stress can be wide-ranging, from the trivial and easily corrected to the serious and potentially difficult to alter. If there are deep-seated problems, the help of a psychiatrist may be needed.

It may be helpful to suggest to the child a **goal** for becoming dry, such as, for example, a weekend camp or an overnight visit to grandparents. Such incentives, however, should be used with caution, as failure will cause further disillusionment.

There are two other forms of treatment that are sometimes suggested, both of which have limited success and are inadvisable.

Restriction of fluids during the day only results in a thirsty child and a more irritable bladder due to concentrated urine. Obviously, a large drink just before bedtime is not a sensible idea, but the child should be allowed to drink as much as desired during the day.

Tricyclic antidepressants have an initial success, but relapse almost invariably occurs once the medication is stopped.

THE FUTURE

Once dry beds have been achieved for a period of several weeks, relapse rarely occurs—except perhaps temporarily at the onset of some infection.

The 1% of children who persist with enuresis into adolescence have difficult problems to overcome. All efforts must be made to ensure that no physical or emotional problems have been missed as a cause for the continuation of enuresis.

Epiglottitis

INCIDENCE

Epiglottitis has become less common since the introduction of a vaccine against its main bacterial cause.

Epiglottitis occurs in children between the ages of 2 and 7 years. The sexes are equally affected.

CAUSATION

Epiglottitis is an upper respiratory tract infection causing inflammation of the epiglottis, the flap of tissue at the back of the throat. This important piece of tissue controls the passage of air into the lungs and the passage of food into the digestive system. Therefore, any swelling of the epiglottis can have far-reaching effects on both breathing and swallowing. In severe cases, the passage of air into the lungs can be completely obstructed.

In the vast majority of cases, the bacterium *Hemophilus influenzae* is the organism responsible for the infection. This organism can be isolated from throat swabs (but see below for the dangers of this procedure), or by blood culture from a child with an acute attack.

CHARACTERISTICS

Epiglottitis has an abrupt onset, and the child will become rapidly ill with:

- a **sore throat;**
- a **fever;**
- **difficulties in swallowing.**

This last symptom is quickly followed by **difficulties in breathing.** In contradistinction from an acute attack of croup, the child's breathing with epiglottis is **quiet and muffled.** (With croup, the breathing is noisy, a condition termed "stridor.") Because of the breathing problems, the child's abdomen contracts with each breath, as can the neck above the collarbone. The contraction is caused by the activity of the accessory muscles of respiration—which are not normally used in breathing. It is only by this means that the child can get sufficient air into the lungs over the swollen and inflamed epiglottis.

Within a few hours, the child will become increasingly ill from the generalized toxic effects of the infection. Speaking is hoarse or impossible, and **drooling** will result from the inability to swallow saliva. Breathing and the pulse rate will rise, and the child will become **exhausted** by the efforts needed to breathe. The child is also **restless** and **anxious**. Sitting up is the preferred position, and the **chin may be poked out** in an attempt to ease breathing.

Sudden **cessation of breathing** can occur as a result of complete blockage of the airway.

MANAGEMENT

Urgent **hospital admission** for pediatric intensive care is vital for a child with a severe attack of epiglottitis. If medical help is not quickly available, a 911 call is necessary. It is important that there is as little upset to the child as possible during the course of this attack. Even a minimal amount of distress can cause the onset of respiratory arrest. Any potentially unpleasant procedures, such as even the simple one of pushing down the tongue to see the throat, should be avoided.

In the hospital, **intubation**—a tube passed down the throat to maintain an open airway—is the first priority. This procedure will also allow the throat to be seen fully, which can confirm the diagnosis—the condition will be obvious when the cherry-red swelling at the base of the tongue is seen.

Intravenous antibiotics will need to be given as soon as possible.

The general condition of the child will also need to be closely **monitored,** as septicemia and/or pneumonia can occur as complications of this unpleasant, and potentially dangerous, disease.

COMPLICATIONS

Pneumonia can follow from epiglottitis. If pneumonia develops, there will be a deterioration of the child's general condition and a cough will become obvious. X-ray examination will show the extent of the problem.

Septicemia—a generalized spread of the infection throughout the body via the bloodstream—is another dangerous possibility, where again the child's general condition will worsen rapidly.

Meningitis can also occur. Headache, vomiting, and stiffness of the child's neck are signs of meningitis that accompany a worsening of the general condition.

These complications all require specific and continuing hospital care.

THE FUTURE

Recovery from an uncomplicated attack of epiglottitis is quick and complete, there being no adverse after-effects.

Epilepsy

ALTERNATIVE NAMES

"Falling sickness"; fits; convulsions; seizures. (The three latter names are frequently used synonymously when discussing the manifestations due to epilepsy, and they will be used interchangeably in the following text.)

INCIDENCE

Epilepsy can be defined as "a recurrent sudden electrical discharge in the brain occurring in the absence of fever." It is this abnormal discharge that produces the typical signs and symptoms of an epileptic seizure. The types of effect seen will depend on which part of the brain is affected. There can be generalized seizures affecting the whole body or partial seizures affecting only certain parts or senses.

In school-age children, the incidence of epilepsy is between 4 and 9 in every 1,000. (In preschool children, febrile convulsions—seen only in children younger than 5 years old—have a different incidence, etiology, and course. These convulsions are the direct effect of a sudden rise in temperature on the immature brain, and they are outgrown by the fifth birthday. The incidence of febrile convulsions is around 3% of all preschool children.)

There are a number of conditions that, at first sight, can closely resemble epilepsy. For example, breath-holding attacks and acute labyrinthitis can closely mimic an epileptic attack. These conditions must be carefully excluded before a diagnosis of epilepsy is made, with all the treatment and restrictions that such a diagnosis can imply.

Epilepsy is known in all countries of the world and affects both sexes.

HISTORY .

Epilepsy has been described since biblical times, and, for many years, society has unjustly stigmatized sufferers from this disorder. Terms such as "demonic" or "mad" have frequently been applied to people suffering from epilepsy. Fortunately, there is now a better understanding of the cause and the course of this condition, and successful drug treatments have been found for the different types of epilepsy. However, continuing

86

further education of the public about—often frightening to witness—epileptic episodes is still necessary.

CAUSATION

Seizures can be part of the symptomatology of complex **syndromes**, such as, for example, Sturge–Weber syndrome and Batten disease. (Approximately 140 genetic disorders associated with seizures have been reported.)

Genetic inheritance appears to have a bearing on the occurrence of primary generalized—or idiopathic—epilepsy. The risk that children of epilepsy sufferers will also have the disorder is estimated to be around 8%.

Developmental abnormalities in the structure of the brain can be the basis of the epilepsy. Some children who show generalized developmental delay can also have seizures as part of the general picture.

Chemical imbalance in the body can give rise to seizures under certain conditions. For example, low calcium or magnesium levels can cause this problem, particularly in newborn babies, as can, under certain circumstances, low blood sugar. Seizures due to these factors cannot be classed as true epilepsy, however, because the abnormal electrical activity will cease once the body physiology has been returned to normal.

Seizures can also be a long-term complication following a **severe head injury.**

Infections, both those occurring prenatally (such as toxoplasmosis or infection with cytomegalovirus) and those occurring later in childhood, can cause epilepsy. Such serious infections as meningitis, septicemia, or encephalitis can leave the child with recurrent seizures following recovery from the acute illness.

Tumors in the brain are another cause of the onset of seizures in a child who has no previous history of epilepsy.

It can be seen that the list of possible causes of seizures is almost as long as the types of seizure themselves. Therefore, great care must be taken to attempt to determine a treatable cause for the seizures before a diagnosis of idiopathic epilepsy is made—with all its future implications for treatment and lifestyle.

CHARACTERISTICS

Generalized seizures

Generalized seizures can be divided into "grand mal," "petit mal," and myoclonic seizures.

Grand mal epilepsy

This type of seizure occurs in about 80% of children who suffer from epilepsy. Before the seizure, the child may behave in an unusual way or be especially irritable for some hours prior to the following sequence of events.

There is a **sudden loss of consciousness** in which the child will fall to the ground and become rigid. At this time, breathing will cease and the child will become blue through lack of oxygen. This is known as the **tonic phase** of a grand mal fit and lasts around 30 seconds.

Following the tonic phase, there will be a phase—known as the **clonic phase**—in which the arms and legs will exhibit jerking movements. This phase is variable in length and can last several minutes. The movements will gradually cease, and the child will slowly regain consciousness, having no memory of the seizure.

Finally, the child may feel the need to **sleep** for a variable length of time, or she or he may be **confused** or **irritable** for a while.

Frothing at the mouth can occur at the height of the seizure, and urinary incontinence may also occur. (Biting of the tongue is an extremely unusual occurrence, in spite of the many lurid stories that abound!)

Petit mal epilepsy

This type of epilepsy can be extremely difficult to diagnose. There are **short periods of altered consciousness** (10–15 seconds only) in which the child stops whatever she or he is doing and stares into space. Following this short period of "absence," the activity or conversation will be picked up again as if there had been no intermission. (Another, descriptive, name for petit mal is "absences.")

These absences can occur many times during the day. Often, the only clue that they are occurring is a decline in the child's school performance. As a result of frequent absences, much can be missed over the course of a day's schooling. If this possibility is remembered, the child can be observed carefully and the attacks noted.

There are no involuntary movements or incontinence during these attacks of petit mal.

Myoclonic seizures

Myoclonic epilepsy most commonly occurs in children who have developmental delay, often due to underlying brain damage. The attacks are brief and may consist of **jerking movements** of arms, body, and/or legs. Occasionally, only the head is involved in the jerky movements. The child may fall to the floor, but she or he will recover quickly. Lennox–Gastaut syndrome—a specialized form of childhood epilepsy—commonly has myoclonic epilepsy as part of its symptomatology.

Partial seizures

There are two main types of partial epileptic seizure. These arise as a result of abnormal electrical discharges in specific parts of the brain.

Rolandic epilepsy (benign partial epilepsy of childhood)

Rolandic epilepsy occurs between the ages of 3 and 12 years. Symptoms occur most frequently at night, or during the period between sleeping and waking. This timing can make diagnosis difficult.

The child is conscious throughout the whole attack. She or he is often unable to speak but will point to the side of the face, obviously trying to convey the unusual feelings that are occurring. During recovery, this area of the face may twitch. The whole episode is over within a couple of minutes.

Occasionally, unusual sensations of swelling or shrinking of an arm or one side of the face can be described afterward by an articulate child.

The electroencephalogram (EEG) in this type of epilepsy shows a very typical diagnostic pattern. Fortunately, this benign type of epilepsy disappears completely around the age of 12 or 13 years, never to reappear. The abnormal EEG tracing gradually returns to normal.

Treatment is rarely necessary, but specific drugs will stop the attacks if they occur too frequently or the child is unduly distressed by them.

Temporal lobe epilepsy

Temporal lobe epilepsy is associated with a number of bizarre symptoms. The child may have specific hallucinations of a visual, auditory, or olfactory nature.

Alternatively, the sufferer may have sudden explosive attacks of rage or intense fear. Objective signs, such as flushing of the face, dilatation of the pupils of the eyes, or perspiration can also occur during an attack.

These occurrences are sometimes followed by a typical grand mal attack. Following the seizure the child feels confused and will need to sleep for an hour or more, although there is no definite memory of the attack.

These attacks are due to a number of possible factors, ranging from a previous severe infection, through a previous lack of oxygen causing damage to a specific part of the brain, to a cerebral tumor.

INVESTIGATIONS

A careful **history** of the attacks is the most important factor in the diagnosis of any form of epilepsy. The sequence of events as well as what actually happened—as described by a witness—will give clues as to whether the attack was epileptic or not.

Tests for chemical imbalances must be done on a sample of blood to exclude such conditions as diabetes or kidney failure, for example.

An **EEG** will show any abnormalities in the brain waves. Many EEG patterns are quite specific for different forms of epilepsy.

CT scans are important follow-up investigations if it is thought that there is some physical abnormality in the brain causing the seizures.

Magnetic resonance imaging may, on occasion, be necessary to demonstrate a tiny lesion that could be missed on a CT scan.

All these investigations must be interpreted in conjunction with a clear account of the actual seizure.

MANAGEMENT

Drugs: The decision to start drug treatment for epilepsy can be a difficult one. Rarely, if ever, are drugs needed for one or two seizures. However, when attacks interfere with a child's everyday activities, drug treatment will be necessary—for example, when there are so many "absences" due to petit mal during a school day that they interfere with the child's ability to learn.

There is a wide range of drugs that can be used to control epilepsy. Each type of epilepsy has a drug, or group of drugs, that will best be able to control the seizures. In order to determine the treatment best suited to each child's individual needs, it may be necessary to try various drugs or combinations of drugs. The most successful drug should then be prescribed on a long-term basis. Most children will need to take the medication twice each day in order to control their seizures adequately. It may be necessary to change the drug regimen as the child matures. Side effects must also be noted, and regular measurements made of blood levels of the drug. Side effects include dizziness, hyperactivity, headache, blurred vision, and learning difficulties. These side effects are quite specific to each drug.

Schooling: Children with epilepsy unrelated to any other pathological condition are quite able to attend an ordinary school. Fifty to seventy percent of children with epilepsy have normal IQs. The remainder of the children probably have a deficit in their intellectual ability due to other problems—which in themselves, of course, have a bearing on the etiology of their seizures.

Teaching staff should be aware of their pupil's problems and be conversant with first aid treatment in case a seizure occurs during the school day. This latter event is, however, unlikely to occur if medication is carefully prescribed—and taken.

Some children will experience **learning difficulties** as a result of their epilepsy or associated disorders. Special schooling for these children will then be necessary.

Activities: Certain activities are dangerous for children with epilepsy. **Swimming** requires the supervision of an adult who, ideally, should be in charge solely of the epileptic child. **Cycling** on the open road in fast-moving traffic should not be allowed. **Gymnastic activities** that necessitate climbing up walls or ropes should be forbidden. Other exercises in the gym are beneficial and should be encouraged.

Other measures include:

Family therapy, following the initial diagnosis, can be helpful if parents are particularly upset regarding the diagnosis. General practitioners, pediatricians, home healthcare workers, and teaching staff can all be involved in helping the family come to terms with the child's epilepsy. What is happening, the purpose of the treatment, and the best ways to help the child live a happy, fulfilled life all need to be explored.

Surgery plays a minor part in the management of epilepsy. This option is restricted to cases of uncontrollable epilepsy in some severely handicapped children.

THE FUTURE

A **driver's license** can be held by an individual with epilepsy, provided that two years have elapsed without a daytime seizure.

Genetic counseling before a pregnancy is undertaken may be necessary for some couples who have a strong family history of epilepsy.

Work: Certain types of employment are inadvisable for people with epilepsy (e.g., work necessitating climbing heights or jobs around continuously moving machinery). Career advice is helpful during the latter years at school.

Cessation of seizures: It has been estimated that between 50% and 70% of children with epilepsy will have no further seizures when they reach adulthood. The outcome in individual cases, of course, is very much dependent upon the type and cause of the epilepsy.

SELF-HELP GROUP

Epilepsy Foundation of America (EFA)
4351 Garden City Drive
Landover, MD 20785-2267
301-459-3700 or 800-332-1000
800-332-2070 TTY

Fifth Disease

ALTERNATIVE NAMES

"Slapped cheek syndrome"; erythema infectiosum.

INCIDENCE

This infection affects children between the ages of 2 and 10 years old. Adults can also be affected, but that is unusual. For some unknown reason, girls are more frequently affected than boys.

Outbreaks of this condition can occur at any time of the year, but they are most common during the winter and the spring. This pattern is in line with the higher incidence of many infections, due to the closer proximity of children to one another, during the colder months of the year.

CAUSATION

Fifth disease is caused by a virus of the parvovirus group. The infection is spread from child to child by droplet infection. The virus is also thought to be contracted from infected blood products when, for example, a child has a blood transfusion. The incubation period reportedly varies from 5 to 20 days after exposure.

CHARACTERISTICS

Frequently, the first sign of "slapped cheek syndrome" is the typical **rash** (similar in type to that seen in rubella) that appears on the child's cheeks. As the name implies, it appears as if the child has received a blow to the face. (Fifth disease must always be remembered as a possibility when there has been a previous high index of suspicion of child abuse.)

In contrast to the bright red rash on the cheeks, the area around the child's mouth is **pale.** (A similar phenomenon is seen in scarlet fever. This latter infection is, however, a far more serious and severe disease, and the two infections are distinguished by the more generalized and serious constitutional symptoms seen in scarlet fever.) In two or three days, the rash extends to the chest and limbs. This rash lasts for a week or two and then gradually fades, but it can reappear for another couple of weeks when the child takes a hot bath. This rash can be mildly irritating.

There may also be a **fever** associated with the illness, usually before the rash appears. Like all feverish illnesses, the raised temperature is associated with **headache** and a general feeling of **malaise** and **aching limbs.**

INVESTIGATIONS

Blood tests: The diagnosis can be confirmed by a specialized laboratory test on a sample of blood. The test is rarely performed in an uncomplicated case of fifth disease, but it may be necessary if any of the rare complications occur.

MANAGEMENT

As with most viral infections, there is no specific treatment, antibiotics being of no value in infections of viral origin.

Analgesics should be given if necessary to control fever, if present to any degree, and to relieve headaches and aching limbs. Dosage must, of course, be appropriate to the age of the child. (Aspirin must not be given to children under the age of 12 years because of the link between this analgesic and Reye syndrome.)

It is not necessary to keep a child with fifth disease away from **school** unless she or he is feeling too unwell due to fever and other symptoms of infection. As infection is passed on from child to child before the rash appears, staying away from school once the rash is present will not help reduce the spread of the infection. Once the rash has appeared, the child is no longer infectious.

COMPLICATIONS

Mild **arthritis** can occur with slapped cheek syndrome, usually beginning a few days before the appearance of the rash. Although this complication more commonly occurs in adults with the infection, children can also suffer. The pain associated with the arthritis tends to come and go in a fleeting fashion, and it can last many weeks. The smaller joints—fingers, wrists, and ankles—are usually affected. Analgesics may be necessary to control this pain.

There are two special groups of children who have complications due to fifth disease. In children who have **thalassemia** or **sickle cell anemia,** the infection may precipitate a "crisis" in which levels of hemoglobin fall dangerously low. Blood transfusion may be necessary for these children until the effects of the virus have worn off. Children with a pre-existing malignancy, particularly **acute leukemia,** can also suffer from complications from fifth disease. Specialized treatment is necessary under these conditions.

PREVENTION

There is no immunization available against slapped cheek syndrome.

THE FUTURE

There is no long-term disability following an attack of fifth disease. The arthritis that sometimes occurs is only temporary and does not recur in later life. If the disease is contracted during pregnancy, miscarriage can occur, but this outcome is not inevitable.

Gastroenteritis

INCIDENCE

Around the world, gastroenteritis is one of the most common of childhood infections. While the incidence of this illness has fallen steadily in the West, gastroenteritis is still one of the major lethal diseases in children in many developing nations. The dramatic fall in fatalities in the West due to this infection has largely been brought about by improved hygiene and the energetic treatment of dehydration in children with an acute attack of gastroenteritis.

Outbreaks of gastroenteritis still occur, however; 50% of the cases occur in children younger than 5 years old. Outbreaks are especially likely in the winter months, when close contact among children is more usual than in the summer months.

HISTORY

Diarrheal diseases have always been a problem when large numbers of people congregate together. Cholera, dysentery, and typhoid were common gastrointestinal disorders prior to the twentieth century. Since that time, public health measures regarding purity of drinking water and disposal of sewage have transformed the picture in developed countries.

CAUSATION

Gastroenteritis can be caused by bacteria or viruses. It is thought that around 50% of all gastroenteritis attacks are caused by the rotavirus. These tiny viruses were first detected in Australia. They can be visualized under the electron microscope.

The infection is probably passed from child to child, particularly when children do not thoroughly wash their hands after using the bathroom. Viral infection can perhaps also be passed on by droplet infection from the respiratory tract—many children with a diarrheal disease have also recently had a cold. Children up to the age of 6 years old are particularly prone to viral forms of gastroenteritis. After that age, the majority of children have built up an immunity to the viruses and so do not suffer from symptoms of the infection.

The Norwalk virus is one of the more publicized viruses causing gastroenteritis in recent years, but there are a number of other viruses which also cause similar unpleasant symptoms.

There are several bacteria that cause gastroenteritis. The most common of these are the *Escherichia coli* (*E. coli*), *Salmonella*, and *Shigella* bacteria. The decline of gastroenteritis cases in the West is largely due to better control of these bacteria. Outbreaks of *Salmonella* still occur, usually due to contaminated food. Contact tracing of these outbreaks is energetically pursued, and appropriate steps are taken to improve hygiene to avoid further problems.

CHARACTERISTICS

Whatever the causative organism, the clinical signs and symptoms of an acute attack of gastroenteritis are similar

The early stages of the infection can well be nonspecific. The baby or young child will be **irritable, cry,** and cease to play happily. Food will be refused, and an excessive thirst may be noticed.

Within a few hours, **vomiting** will occur, especially in younger children. Vomiting will usually precede the **diarrhea,** which soon follows. (These symptoms can also, of course, occur in other conditions, which need surgery—for example, appendicitis and intussusception.) **Fever** is variable—sometimes only a mild fever is present, while at other times the temperature is high. A high fever occurs more frequently with an infection by the rotavirus group.

INVESTIGATIONS

Usually—and fortunately—attacks of gastroenteritis in children are short-lived and mild. In these cases, no investigation into the causative organism is necessary. However, if an outbreak occurs in a nursery or a school, for example, samples of the stools of sufferers and their families should be sent to the laboratory for identification of the infecting organism.

MANAGEMENT

Toddlers and older children

In **mild cases** where vomiting and frequent diarrhea are not a serious problem, **fluids only** should be given for 24 hours. With the young child, this restriction is not usually a problem, as food is the last thing she or he will wish to see or take! Plain water, or water with the addition of a tea-spoon of glucose to a glass, whenever the child complains of thirst is all that is necessary for 24 hours. Following this period, provided that vomiting has ceased and the diarrhea has improved, solid food can be reintroduced gradually over the next few days.

In more severe cases, **replacement of lost fluid** by one of the commercial replacement fluids (obtainable from pharmacies) will be necessary. Again, no solid food should be given.

Medical advice should always be sought if the diarrhea and vomiting are severe and/or persist for longer than a few hours. Such advice is especially important for young children. Large amounts of fluid can be lost by severe diarrhea and vomiting, and small children cannot easily replace this loss.

Hospital admission may be necessary for the small child with a severe attack of gastroenteritis, because of this fluid loss. Under these circumstances, not only is the loss of fluid itself potentially dangerous but the blood chemistry can be seriously disarranged. Skilled medical and nursing care are required.

Babies under 1 year old

Similar treatment is necessary for small babies as for older children, but it must be remembered that tiny babies become dehydrated very quickly and can become dangerously ill in a very short time. Therefore, medical advice must be obtained quickly for these little ones.

Kaolin, or any of the other anti-diarrheal agents, is of no value in childhood gastroenteritis.

Antibiotics are also of no value in gastroenteritis due to a virus, but they should be used in proven cases of *Salmonella* infection.

COMPLICATIONS

Dehydration, as described above, is the most immediate and serious complication.

Sugar intolerance is a common complication following an attack of gastroenteritis. The younger the child, the more frequently this problem occurs. Symptoms appear as soon as milk is reintroduced into the diet following the initial treatment. Diarrhea will again become a problem, with frequent, frothy, watery stools that in turn often give rise to an unpleasant diaper rash. (It is the lactose in the milk that causes the diarrhea.) The basic cause of this temporary intolerance is the damage done to the lining of the intestine by the bacteria or virus causing the gastroenteritis.

Treatment is to give a lactose-free milk for a few weeks to allow the intestine time to recover. After about four to six weeks, ordinary milk should be gradually reintroduced into the diet; usually there is no return of the diarrhea. If there diarrhea does recur, the process should be repeated until ordinary milk is tolerated again.

PREVENTION

It would be ideal if all attacks of gastroenteritis in children—and adults—could be prevented. Unfortunately, it is difficult to imagine this scenario, although work is proceeding toward a vaccine against the rotavirus.

Good hygiene in the preparation of food and regular hand-washing after visiting the toilet and before meals are important ways to control the spread of infection.

Medical advice should be obtained sooner, rather than later, especially in the case of young babies, in order to prevent complications.

Hand, Foot, and Mouth Disease

INCIDENCE

Small outbreaks of this graphically named infection can occur among babies and older children. The summer months are the most likely time for the condition to occur. Adults can suffer from the disease as well as children.

HISTORY

Hand, foot, and mouth disease was first recognized as a clinical entity in Toronto in 1957. An outbreak of the infection occurred with quite specific features, and it was named according to the characteristics noted. (The name bears an unfortunate resemblance to the foot and mouth disease found in cattle, but the conditions are absolutely unrelated.)

CAUSATION

Hand, foot, and mouth disease is caused by a virus of the Coxsackie group. The virus can be isolated from the skin lesions and also from the stools of sufferers.

The incubation period for this infection is unknown.

CHARACTERISTICS

There may be a mild constitutional upset before the typical rash appears. The child may have a **mild fever,** and she or he may complain of a **headache** and a general feeling of **malaise.**

Babies may be reluctant to take their feedings, and older children be unwilling to eat as the rash starts to make its appearance.

The **rash** is very specific, consisting of small, grayish-white, blistered spots with a surrounding red halo. These are found on the tongue, making this mobile organ sore. The palms of the hands and the sides of the soles of the feet are also affected. Occasionally, this rash may become more widespread, most often covering the buttocks, although other parts of the body may be affected as well. (If the rash does occur on the buttocks, confusion can arise between this condition and Henoch–Schönlein purpura.)

The rash lasts between three and five days and then fades rapidly. Other symptoms, if present, then also improve rapidly, and the child is restored to full health.

MANAGEMENT

General sympathetic care is all that is required for an attack of hand, foot, and mouth disease. **Fluids only** for a day or two may be required if the child's mouth is sore following the appearance of the rash. Otherwise, **bland foods** will be better tolerated than spicy, highly flavored ones until the tongue has returned to normal.

Analgesics to reduce fever and relieve headache should be given if necessary. Only acetaminophen compounds should be given to children, as aspirin increases the risk, in under-12-year-olds, of Reye syndrome.

School-age children should **remain away from school** while the rash is present on their hands. As the incubation period of this infection is unknown, the time when it can be passed on is uncertain, but, as with most viral infections, the most infectious period is probably the time just before the rash appears.

COMPLICATIONS

The only complication that has been reported to occur with this infection is the **extension of the rash all over the body.** This complication is rare, but it must be remembered when a child is seen with a rash that covers the whole of the body. The diagnosis can be made by the very obvious grayish rash that covers the palms of the hands and soles of the feet.

THE FUTURE

There are no long-term effects in later life from hand, foot, and mouth disease.

Hay Fever

ALTERNATIVE NAME

Seasonal allergic rhinitis.

INCIDENCE

It is thought that between 10 and 20% of the population suffer from hay fever. The time of the year at which the symptoms appear depends upon which particular tree or flower produces the allergy in each individual person.

Springtime—March to May—when many plants come into bloom shows the highest incidence of hay fever. Late flowering plants such as carnations, dahlias, and chrysanthemums, as well as ragweed, can all produce symptoms later in the year, from July to September. Molds and mildews, usually at their height during warm, damp weather, can also affect some people. Therefore, while hay fever is at its height during the spring, certain sufferers are not immune for the rest of the year.

Hay fever affects both sexes equally and even young children can be affected, although most children first begin to suffer during the early school years.

It has been reported that children of non-manual workers are more prone to hay fever.

CAUSATION

Hay fever is the third member of the allergy trio: asthma, eczema, and hay fever. The cause is an allergic reaction to the pollens of many different types of trees, grasses, and flowers. The amount of pollen produced by just one flower is incredible—a single sorrel blossom can produce 180,000 grains of pollen, and in a high wind, these grains can be carried for more than ten miles! It is difficult indeed to avoid contact with these minute grains of pollen.

Susceptibility to these allergens is often inherited. Other members of the family may not themselves suffer from hay fever, but they may have asthma or eczema.

Symptoms, of course, are at their worst when the pollen count is high.

CHARACTERISTICS

Profuse clear, watery **discharge from the nose,** often associated with sneezing, is typical.

Red, runny, itchy eyes, sometimes known by the alternative name of "allergic conjunctivitis," can occur without the other symptoms of hay fever. The causative factors are similar.

Wheezing and **breathlessness** can occur with hay fever as well as with asthma. The differential diagnosis between these two conditions can at times be blurred.

Itching of the soft palate and/or the ears, due to a common nerve supply between these two structures, can be a symptom.

Diagnosis is based on the occurrence of these symptoms at times of the year that are specific to each sufferer.

MANAGEMENT

It is virtually impossible to avoid contact with pollen altogether. Even if that were possible, it would be hard to keep children indoors during the warm summer months. There are a number of drug treatments available that will subdue most of the symptoms of hay fever.

Eyedrops of sodium cromoglycate—the same drug that is used as a prophylactic measure in asthma—are very successful in keeping the eye symptoms under control. The drops will need to be instilled on a regular basis four times a day. This regimen must be strictly followed throughout the hay fever season.

Antihistamines (there are those available that do not cause drowsiness) are helpful for mild cases, and again should be used throughout the season.

Steroids used in an inhaler are necessary for more severe cases.

Steroids given orally in tablet form can be used in the short term for children with disabling symptoms of hay fever. These drugs (which are not advised for long-term use) are useful to tide a teenager with severe hay fever over a difficult examination period, for example.

THE FUTURE

Some sufferers find that their hay fever improves as the years go by, but most children suffering from hay fever will continue to do so throughout their lives. It is fortunate that there are drugs available to control the symptoms. In older children that have intractable symptoms that do not abate with age, allergy shots are a consideration. However, shots require a commitment of several years duration for injections that may need to be given as frequently as once a week.

Headache

INCIDENCE

Headaches are a surprisingly common symptom in children. By the age of 10 years, it is thought that around 10% of all children have headaches of a recurring nature. Another study of children younger than 5 years old found that 19% had complained of a headache. (Young children often do not have the verbal skills to describe their pain, but comments such as "my head is sore" or "my head bangs" are common, while other children show their distress by holding their heads or burying them in a pillow.)

Headaches are often part and parcel of other illnesses, the associated symptoms of which override the pain of the headache. For example, the fever and rash of an infectious childhood illness, such as chicken pox, will take precedence over the headache, although the headache is undoubtedly present.

CAUSATION

Headaches can be divided into three main causative groups:

- **vascular** (related to the blood system) **headaches**—migraine is the classical example of this type of headache;
- **"tension" headaches;**
- **headaches associated with other illnesses.** This last group can be further subdivided into those headaches that have an infection as their prime cause and those due to other problems, such as brain tumors or previous head injury.

There is another small subgroup of conditions that can give rise to pain which children can describe as a "headache." Such conditions include sinusitis and visual difficulties, such as untreated near-sightedness.

Headaches in children are a worrying symptom for parents. At the back of everyone's mind is the thought of serious conditions, such as a brain tumor or meningitis. While these conditions are comparatively rare reasons for a headache, medical advice should be sought sooner rather than later, particularly if the headache is severe, if it lasts longer than three to four hours, or if it is associated with other symptoms, such as vomiting and/or fever.

CHARACTERISTICS

Vascular headaches are those that cause migraines. This condition is fully described in the entry on migraine.

Tension headaches have different characteristics from those of migraine. They tend to be more continuous, not occurring in definite episodes as does a migraine. The headache is usually **present every day** and often **persists throughout the day** at varying levels of pain or discomfort.

Headaches of this type are not usually as severe as the pain of a full-blown attack of migraine. Children often describe this type of headache as a tight **band around the head.** Also, pain in the muscles at the **back of the neck** can be a feature. Unlike migraine, there is no visual disturbance or vomiting.

With this type of headache, it is worth making inquiries into the child's activities and behavior at daycare or school. A specific **learning difficulty** or other worrying aspect of school life, such as **bullying,** can be the basic cause of this type of headache.

Children, as well as adults, can suffer from **depression**—perhaps more frequently than is realized. Marital discord, stepfamily difficulties, and bereavement over the death of a close family member can all be sources of depression, which can be manifested as a tension headache. Other more subtle reasons, such as fear of the dark or a worrying television program, for example, must be remembered when attempting to sort out the cause of a tension headache.

Headaches associated with other illnesses can again be subdivided into three distinct categories.

Those infectious illnesses—influenza, a common cold, or chicken pox, for example—that involve a **fever** are all associated to some degree with headaches. This symptom may be one of the child's least concerns when all limbs ache, his/her entire body is hot and sticky, and, to add to the miseries, an itchy rash appears! Nevertheless, if questioned specifically, the presence of a headache will be noted.

More seriously, there are those headaches that are caused by **brain tumors.** Under these circumstances the headache is usually **worse in the mornings** when the child wakes. **Sleep** may also have been disturbed by the pain of the headache—in fact, the mere act of lying down can at times worsen the pain. Headaches due to this cause tend to be **continuous,** with exacerbation of the severity of the pain under the conditions mentioned. There may be other signs of the underlying problem, such as some specific **muscle weakness** or **double vision,** depending on the actual position of the tumor. **Seizures** can occur, as can subtle changes in **personality** or **behavior.**

Headaches can also occur some time after a **head injury** in which bleeding has occurred beneath one particular layer of the membranes covering the brain. The subsequent blood clot—known as a **subdural hematoma**—will press on the surrounding tissue, giving rise to a headache. Dangerous further **bleeding** can occur at a later date under these circumstances.

If any of these conditions is suspected, further investigations—a **scan** and possibly **magnetic resonance imaging**—will be urgently required. Following the results of these tests, appropriate treatment—surgical or chemical—will need to be instituted.

MANAGEMENT

Basically, the treatment of a headache must address the underlying cause, with the addition of a drug such as **acetaminophen**—in appropriate dosage for the child's age—to subdue the pain until specific treatment can be given.

Tension headaches need careful and sympathetic investigation into the possible source of **stress.** As previously mentioned, inquiries need to be made into any problems—whether related to learning or social contact—arising at school. Children are often reluctant to tell parents of difficulties that they may be having at school—if indeed they are even aware of what exactly is the matter. At times, the help of an **educational psychologist** will need to be enlisted if learning difficulties are a possibility.

It is counter-productive to keep a child with a tension headache away from **school.** Lessons will be missed, causing extra stress when they have to be made up. It also important to ensure that both child and parents know that tension headaches are not serious and not an indication of any sinister disease.

Headaches due to intercurrent illness, such as a cold or flu, will improve once the disease has run its course. Acetaminophen will help reduce the pain of the associated headache, as well as lowering temperature and improving the pain of aching limbs.

Headaches due to brain tumors or subdural hematoma need special investigations and treatments appropriate to each individual case.

To summarize, headaches in children need **further investigation** if:

- the headache is **worse in the mornings** when awakening from sleep;
- the headache is worse when the child **coughs;**
- the headache **wakes** the child or **prevents sleep;**

- there is **weakness, numbness, or tingling** in any part of the body in association with the headache;
- persistent **vomiting** occurs with the headache;
- there is any **change in the child's personality or behavior.**

Henoch–Schönlein Purpura

ALTERNATIVE NAME

Anaphylactoid purpura.

INCIDENCE

There are no available figures for this condition, but it is not an especially common disorder. Nevertheless, when it does occur, the signs and symptoms are sufficiently severe to cause alarm and—at times—difficulties in diagnosis.

Henoch–Schönlein purpura can run a protracted course, with associated implications for both care and education. Fortunately, full recovery—in a time scale ranging from six weeks to one year—is the usual outcome of this disease.

The condition is most common among preschool children, even as young as one year old, but all age groups can be affected.

Boys are more frequently affected than girls.

HISTORY

The double-barreled name of this disease arose due to the involvement of two doctors—Henoch and Schönlein—in the description of the condition. Henoch described the relationship of the specific rash with the gastrointestinal symptoms, while Schönlein placed emphasis on the relationship of the rash with the arthritic manifestations. It was later realized that both descriptions related to the one disease.

CAUSATION

The basic cause of Henoch–Schönlein purpura is unknown, but it probably results from an immune system problem.

The pathology is one of inflammation around the capillaries and small arteries (a vasculitis) in many—and varied—parts of the body, including the skin, the gastrointestinal tract, and the kidneys.

There have been suggestions that the onset of the condition may be preceded by an upper respiratory tract infection, but that is not always the case.

CHARACTERISTICS

The typical **rash** is usually the first sign of the disease. This rash consists of small, bruise-like ("purpuric") spots around a blistered center. This rash, unlike a number of other rashes, does not disappear when pressed with a finger. It is the result of the inflammatory process around the blood vessels.

The distribution of the rash is quite distinctive, being mainly confined to the backs of the legs and the buttocks. In some children, the rash may be minimal and confined to only a few spots. But if the few spots are seen in a child who complains of the other typical symptoms, the diagnosis is clear.

The rash is painless and does not itch. As fading takes place over the succeeding days, the typical yellow discoloration seen on a fading bruise is seen.

Gastrointestinal tract: symptoms in this body system are often the most unpleasant aspects of Henoch–Schönlein purpura. Because of the lesions—similar to the ones seen on the skin—in the intestine, bleeding occurs. The bleeding gives rise to **colicky abdominal pain,** which can either be persistent or come and go intermittently. Acute abdominal pain in children is notoriously difficult to diagnose, as there are a multitude of possible causes. It is the relationship of the pain with the skin rash that provides the clue to the diagnosis of Henoch–Schönlein purpura. **Vomiting** can also occur in association with the abdominal pain.

Blood in the bowel movements is a common feature, although the blood may not be obvious to the naked eye. Laboratory testing will confirm that bleeding into the intestine has occurred.

Children with this kind of continuing abdominal pain will often become unduly **depressed**—understandably so. There is nothing quite so lowering to the spirits as a continuing stomach ache.

Joints: Some joints of the body can be affected. The child will complain of **pain** and **tenderness,** particularly on movement. This pain, like the abdominal pain, can be intermittent. This symptom is due to the inflammation of the small blood vessels around the affected joints.

Renal tract: The kidneys can also be specifically involved in Henoch–Schönlein purpura. Renal problems are an especially worrying aspect of this otherwise benign disease, as long-term effects can result from the involvement of the renal tract. Similar to the problems affecting the gastrointestinal tract, there can be bleeding from the small blood vessels in the renal tract. Blood in the urine may not be visible to the naked eye, but it can be demonstrated by laboratory testing. Along with the blood, microscopic amounts of protein are present in the urine, again demonstrable in the laboratory.

The timing of the renal tract involvement can be unusual, occasionally arising as late as three months after the appearance of the rash. Therefore, it is important that a check should be kept on the child's urine at intervals for several months after an attack of Henoch–Schönlein purpura. (In a few—very rare—cases, the kidney involvement is a major feature of the disease, running a rapidly downhill course ending in fatal renal failure.)

Henoch–Schönlein purpura is a condition that can resolve completely within six weeks, leaving the child in complete health. However, there can also be relapses, with abdominal and joint pain recurring for as long as one year and protein continuing to be excreted in the urine, showing that the kidneys are still being affected by the disease. In the vast majority of cases, recovery is eventually complete, with no long-lasting ill effects.

INVESTIGATIONS

Blood tests show few specific changes in an attack of Henoch–Schönlein purpura.

Urine tests, as mentioned, show varying amounts of protein and/ or blood, indicating the degree to which the kidneys are involved in the condition.

MANAGEMENT

Although there are no specific drugs that will produce a dramatic cure, careful management of the—sometimes very distressing—symptoms of the disease is important.

Bed rest during the period when the rash is at its height is advised. It has been found that the rash tends to worsen if the child is allowed to run around. Also, if there is obvious bleeding from the renal tract, bed rest is advisable.

Analgesics to control the pain from tender joints will give much relief. The abdominal pain can also be controlled by analgesics. In mild cases, acetaminophen will suffice, but children with severe abdominal pain will need stronger drugs to control this distressing symptom. Occasionally, steroids will be needed to give relief.

Emotional support for both parents and child during the possibly long-drawn-out process of this disease is important. Full explanations of the possible cause and probable sequence of events should be given, so that parents can cope with each new manifestation if, or when, it arises. The child's possible depression also needs to be discussed, and plans made to mitigate this problem as far as possible.

Schooling can be resumed when the rash has disappeared and pain is absent from joints. Because of the possibility of relapses, teachers should be kept advised of problems as they arise. Work may need to be sent home if the child is not up to coping with the rough and tumble of the school day. School staff should also be reassured that the condition is not infectious.

Regular **review of kidney function,** together with blood pressure measurements, should be done until all signs of protein in the urine are absent.

COMPLICATIONS

The important complication of continuing renal involvement must always be borne in mind. **Hypertension** (high blood pressure) can result from severe involvement of the kidneys. If it occurs, it should be treated to avoid further problems in later life.

Nephrotic syndrome, in which there is continuing, and excessive, amounts of protein excreted in the urine, together with marked swelling of various of parts of the body, can also—but rarely—result from an attack of Henoch–Schönlein purpura.

THE FUTURE

Henoch–Schönlein purpura is rarely fatal. However, if renal involvement has been severe, high blood pressure may be a problem in later life.

Impetigo

INCIDENCE

Impetigo is a well-known skin disease that affects people worldwide. In the past decade, there has been an increase in the type of impetigo caused by a specific bacterium, *Staphylococcus*, with a decrease in impetigo caused by other bacteria.

Children are especially prone to this skin infection.

CAUSATION

Impetigo can be caused by either *Staphylococcus* or *Streptococcus* bacteria. As mentioned above, there has been a worldwide increase lately in impetigo caused by *Staphylococci*. Streptococcal impetigo is rarely seen nowadays. The type of bacteria involved has a bearing on the type of treatment necessary to cure the infection.

Impetigo often arises following other skin diseases such as eczema, scabies, or even a minor insect bite. Scratching induced by these other skin conditions allows the bacteria to enter the abraded surface of the skin.

CHARACTERISTICS

Impetigo is an infection of the skin. Initially, a **small, blistered spot** appears. The area around the mouth and nose is most frequently affected, although theoretically any part of the body can be affected. The skin in the former areas is more liable to infection because of the general soreness and irritation, with subsequent rubbing, caused by the common cold.

The initial sore spot increases, with sometimes alarming rapidity, both in size and in the number of lesions.

Within a few hours, the surface of the skin breaks down, leaving a raw, moist surface that quickly becomes crusted over. In a particular subtype of impetigo, much serum is exuded from the broken-down rash, forming a thick, yellow crust over an underlying reddened, sore area.

Impetigo is a highly contagious condition. In spite of the alarming sight of the rash of impetigo, this infection is **neither painful nor itchy,** and there is rarely any associated generalized systemic upset.

As the rash clears following treatment, superficial skin cells can sometimes be shed, leaving a raw area for a short time. This condition is known as "scalded skin syndrome" or **Lyell disease.** The rash of impetigo fortunately leaves no permanent scarring.

INVESTIGATIONS

Ideally, a swab should be taken from an open lesion and sent to the laboratory so that the invading organism can be identified. With this information, the most suitable antibiotic can then be prescribed. Identification of the bacteria is especially important if a number of children—in a classroom for example—are involved, or if the treatment given is not proving to be successful.

MANAGEMENT

As impetigo is caused by bacteria, **antibiotics** will soon clear the unpleasant rash. While results of the tests identifying the particular organism are awaited (or if no swab has been taken), erythromycin, given by mouth, is one of the most useful antibiotics. In early stages, or in cases where only a small area of skin is involved, an antibiotic cream may be sufficient to produce a cure.

School, and contact with other children, **should be avoided** until the lesions have completely cleared. Because of its highly infectious nature, impetigo can spread like wildfire around a class of schoolchildren or a daycare center. Infection is particularly likely among the younger age groups, partly because of their incomplete knowledge of hygiene at this age!

COMPLICATIONS

On the rare occasions that the group A *Streptococcus* bacterium is the cause of the impetigo, watch should be kept, for around two months after the infection, for possible **kidney involvement.** Signs of renal problems will be:

- blood in the urine;
- swelling of tissues, particularly around the face;
- a decrease in the amount of urine passed.

This condition is serious, and it must receive urgent treatment. It must be stressed, however, that this development is extremely rare—especially as impetigo due to streptococcal bacteria is unusual these days.

Impetigo may complicate a pre-existing eczema.

THE FUTURE

There are no long-term after-effects of an uncomplicated attack of impetigo. The condition can recur, as immunity to the bacteria is not gained by the one attack.

Intussusception

INCIDENCE

Intussusception is a condition primarily seen in infancy, 3 to 9 months old being the most usual age for this condition to occur. It can occur in older children, but the reasons for intussusception in those cases are usually different from the reasons behind cases occurring in infancy.

Some authorities report that the incidence is markedly higher in boys than in girls—the ratio being as high as 5:1. Other professionals consider the incidence to be the same in both sexes.

Intussusception has been described in all races.

CAUSATION

Although the cause cannot be definitely stated in each individual case, it is thought that changes in the content of the bowel during the transition from nursing to solid food may be a causative factor in the younger age group.

In older children, an intussusception can be due to a cyst or a polyp on the bowel, a Meckel's diverticulum (a small duct abnormally present from embryological days), or a hemorrhage into the bowel wall due to some other condition such as leukemia or Henoch–Schönlein purpura.

In both age groups, the cause may be enlargement of specific areas of lymphoid tissue in the bowel as the result of an infectious process.

HISTORY

In 1898, Sir Frederick Treves first described the actual events in the bowel that result in an intussusception. He accurately described the invagination of a part of the bowel into the lumen of another adjacent part. The initial onset of an intussusception can be due to any number of factors (as discussed above).

CHARACTERISTICS

Colicky abdominal pain is the first sign of an intussusception. Knees are drawn up, and the baby becomes **pale** as the pain heightens. There may initially be some period of time between these attacks of pain, but as the condition worsens, the bouts of colic become more frequent.

Vomiting, due to obstruction of the bowel, follows the abdominal pain.

Diarrhea, with the "red currant" stools, occurs later. Not all babies show this feature, so diagnosis must not be delayed because of this omission.

A sausage-shaped **swelling** can be felt in between bouts of colic, usually on the right-hand side of the baby's abdomen or across the top of the abdomen just below the ribs. (The position of the swelling will, of course, vary according to where the intussusception has occurred.)

INVESTIGATIONS

An **X-ray** of the abdomen will show the location of the obstruction by demonstrating abnormal fluid levels in the bowel.

Ultrasound will also show the position of the intussusception and is usually the preferred investigation.

MANAGEMENT

If the baby is seriously ill and dehydrated, rehydration with **intravenous fluids** will be necessary before any attempt is made to reduce the intussusception. If vomiting has been a prominent feature, a **nasogastric tube** will need to be put in place to remove the contents of the stomach.

Reduction of the intussusception, i.e., the putting back in place of the invaginated bowel (rather like turning an inside-out sleeve right side out), can be done in two ways:

- nonsurgically, by the use of a **barium enema** under radiological control. This procedure involves running warm diluted barium into the bowel through a special catheter (with the baby fully sedated). The passage of the barium is watched on the X-ray screen until the position of the intussusception is reached. By the continuing pressure of the column of barium, the invaginated bowel can be pushed back into its normal position. Air, instead of the barium mixture, can also be used successfully to reduce an intussusception. (In China, the air method has been used successfully for centuries—fire-bellows being used to force the air into the bowel!)
- **surgically,** if the nonsurgical method has been found to be unsuccessful. The baby is anesthetized, and the intussusception is

reduced by hand. Occasionally, a part of the bowel will need to be removed because it is damaged. One advantage of the surgical method is that the appendix is usually removed at the same time, which removes the possibility of appendicitis in later life.

THE FUTURE

In very rare instances, a second intussusception can occur, regardless of the method of treatment has been used.

There are no adverse sequelae in later life.

Kawasaki Disease

ALTERNATIVE NAME

Mucocutaneous lymph node syndrome.

INCIDENCE

Kawasaki disease is seen in all parts of the world, but persons of Asian descent have the highest incidence. This disease occurs almost exclusively in young children, around 80% of cases being seen in children under the age of 4 years old. The end of the first year of life seems to be the most usual time for the condition to occur. It is rarely seen in children older than 8 years old.

It is thought that only around 2 children in every 100,000 are affected. Even though Kawasaki disease is a comparatively rare condition in the Western world, it is vital that the condition is recognized and treated appropriately because of the later complications that can occur.

HISTORY

Kawasaki disease, with more than 80,000 reported occurrences, was first described in Japan by Dr. Tamisaku Kawasaki about 25 years ago. In Japan, epidemics have occurred, with a 3-year cycle. These epidemics occur more frequently in winter and early spring. In the United States, no cyclical pattern has been noticed and the disease is seen more often in the spring.

CAUSATION

The cause of Kawasaki disease remains, at present, a mystery. From epidemiological studies and certain features of the disease, the cause would appear to be an infectious one. However, even using modern techniques, it has not proved possible to unearth a specific bacterial or viral organism responsible. Work is proceeding on the possibility that a toxin with a specific action on the immune system is the underlying cause.

While Kawasaki disease has occurred in epidemics—at least in Japan—there is little evidence of transmission from one child to another. There is also little to suggest that the disease has a genetic basis, although the high susceptibility of Asian children suggests that there may be a genetic predisposition to the condition.

CHARACTERISTICS

The characteristics of this unusual, but potentially dangerous, disease are variable. Diagnosis is dependent upon recognition of the clinical signs and symptoms, as there is no specific laboratory test for Kawasaki disease.

Fever is a constant feature, and in the early stages of the disease, it can be the only abnormality. The child's temperature will be high, with spikes of even higher fever. The high fever can continue for up to two weeks, and the child may have a low-grade fever for another two or three weeks.

There are a number of other signs and symptoms characterizing Kawasaki disease, and, for a positive diagnosis, at least four of the following conditions need to be present.

A **rash** appears within one week of the onset of the fever, and it is very variable in appearance. It can resemble the rash of scarlet fever or that of measles, while at other times the urticarial rash of hives can be seen.

Conjunctivitis—a reddening of the "white" part of the eye without any obvious pus formation—can be seen soon after the beginning of the fever. As with the fever, this feature can remain for up to two weeks.

Dryness and redness of the **lips, tongue,** and **throat** can occur. Lips can crack and even bleed in severe cases.

Signs in **fingers and toes** are a fairly constant sign of Kawasaki disease. Palms of the hands and soles of the feet become reddened and swollen. After around 10 to 14 days, the skin will begin to peel from these extremities.

Lymph glands in the neck are often swollen and tender, although this feature is only seen in about half the children with this disease.

Along with these specific signs and symptoms will be the general irritability and loss of appetite associated with a high temperature, from whatever cause.

It is important that other conditions with somewhat similar symptoms (including various bacterial infections of the throat, as well as measles and scarlet fever) are excluded as possible diagnoses.

The child will be acutely ill during the initial two weeks of the illness. After that time, the fever will lessen (although the child will frequently continue to have a low-grade fever); the rash will disappear; and swelling in the lymph nodes will subside. Around that time, the skin will peel from hands and feet. Also at that time, the child may complain of aching joints.

The most serious aspect of Kawasaki disease is the possible involvement of the **heart and coronary arteries.** This complication is thought to occur in between 20 and 30% of children. Signs of heart and/or coronary artery problems arise within the first ten days of the illness. **Chest pain** and **pulse irregularities** can occur as well as other signs of heart failure—**breathlessness** and **swollen feet and ankles.** These difficulties generally resolve with appropriate treatment. Occasionally, however, permanent damage can be done to the coronary arteries when an aneurysm (a ballooning) forms in one of the tiny blood vessels that supply the heart muscle with vital oxygen. This aneurysm can rupture, or the heart muscle can become so starved of oxygen that a "heart attack" is the fatal outcome. This tragic scenario is uncommon, but it must always be remembered as a remote possibility.

INVESTIGATIONS

Blood tests give useful, but unspecific, information. There is often an associated abnormality in the platelets (the part of the blood concerned with the regulation of clotting mechanisms).

Echocardiography is advisable when the diagnosis of Kawasaki disease is certain. This test will show any heart involvement that has occurred and should be repeated six weeks after the onset of the illness.

MANAGEMENT

Aspirin is the mainstay of treatment in Kawasaki disease. It acts by lowering temperature and helps prevent the platelets in the blood from clumping together. (Because aspirin may play a part in causing Reye syndrome, it is usually not recommended for children under the age of 12 years. However, with Kawasaki disease, the benefits of aspirin in preventing heart damage outweigh this remote risk.) High doses of aspirin are necessary for the first week of the disease. A lower dose of aspirin is then given until approximately six weeks have passed since the onset of the disease, when the possibility of heart damage—monitored by echocardiography—is eliminated.

Intravenous doses of **gammaglobulin** have been used in clinical trials in the USA and Japan and have been shown to lessen the risk of heart involvement. This treatment is generally reserved for children who already have some form of heart disease or those children who are at high risk of heart involvement (most usually babies under the age of 1 year with a severe attack of Kawasaki disease).

Another drug that acts on the platelets can be used as an alternative to aspirin or gammaglobulin can be used. The appropriate treatment will need to be decided for each individual child.

General care with sufficient **rest,** a **light diet,** and **plenty of fluids** will be needed during the acute phase of the illness, and a sufficiently **long convalescent period** is necessary to ensure that there has been no heart damage.

THE FUTURE

The future outlook will obviously depend on whether or not heart involvement has occurred. Without this complication, there are no known after-effects from an attack of Kawasaki disease.

SELF-HELP GROUP

Kawasaki Families' Network
46-111 Nahewai Place
Kaneohe, HI 96744
808-525-8053
http://ourworld.compuserve.com/homepages/kawasaki
email: kawasaki@compuserve.com

Lazy Eye

ALTERNATIVE NAME

Strabismus.

INCIDENCE

Lazy eye in children is not a disease entity comparable to, for example, an infectious condition or a congenital problem, but early treatment of this condition is vital if full vision is to be preserved.

The exact incidence of lazy eye in children is not documented. It is thought that around 50% of children who have a lazy eye are related to someone else who has the same condition. The lazy eye itself is not directly inherited, but factors associated with the production of the lazy eye can be passed from generation to generation. In view of this finding, it is important that the brothers and sisters of a child with a lazy eye should also be examined for this condition.

It is especially important to diagnose those children in whom the lazy eye is not immediately obvious. Slight or latent lazy eyes can have as great a deleterious effect on good binocular vision as can a more obvious lazy eye.

Lazy eye can occur in any axis of the eye, but by far the most common types of lazy eye are the **convergent** type (in which one eye turns inward) and the **divergent** type (in which one eye turns outward).

For the first few weeks of life, before muscle coordination is fully developed, all babies can have lazy eyes. Any lazy eye in a baby older than 4 months should be investigated.

CAUSATION

There are a number of conditions that can be factors in the etiology of a lazy eye.

A **refractive error in one eye** is by far the most common cause of a lazy eye. Under these circumstances, one eye focuses more clearly on objects at particular distances than does the other eye. For example, a convergent lazy eye can occur when one eye focuses more clearly than the other on an object a great distance away; in this case, each eye sees an image that is distinct from that seen by the other. (This condition is known as hypermetropia.) To blend the two perceived objects into one image, the muscles in the farsighted eye will accommodate by pulling that eye further inward than the other. Conversely, a nearsighted (myopic) eye—focusing clearly on close objects—will need less accommodation, and so a divergent lazy eye will be the result.

Injuries to the cornea, resulting in scarring of this external sensitive part of the eye, can also give rise to a lazy eye.

The onset of a lazy eye in a child who did not previously have the condition can be the first clue to **diseases of the retina or optic nerve,** such as, for example, a retinoblastoma.

Occlusion of one eye by a pad or bandage, following some injury to an eye or the face, can cause a lazy eye to develop in a surprisingly short time. The covered eye will become amblyopic (non-seeing), through disuse. Treatment to reverse this process must be undertaken with a degree of urgency to prevent permanent loss of vision in the affected eye.

While a simple refractive error is the most common cause of a lazy eye, the other possible factors must always be borne in mind.

CHARACTERISTICS

Lazy eyes, as mentioned previously, come in a variety of guises—convergent or divergent and also, to a much lesser extent, in the vertical axis. Children with lazy eye in the vertical axis will often tilt their heads to compensate for the lazy eye—a useful clue that a lazy eye may be present in cases where the condition is not immediately obvious.

Lazy eye can also be alternating in character (i.e., one eye is fixed on an object at one time, only to be quickly followed by the other eye being fixed on the object instead). In this condition, true binocular vision (in which the two eyes fix and focus on one object to produce one image) is never achieved.

Lazy eye can cause two images to be seen, although there is only one object present (double vision). To compensate for this condition, the part of the brain concerned with vision will suppress one of these images—for example, the image seen by the lazy eye—and as a result, the eye will eventually lose all ability to see. This condition is known as **amblyopia.** It is to prevent this loss of vision in one eye that early intervention in lazy eye is vital, because the lack of vision can become permanent if treatment is not given.

Lazy eye can be very obvious, even to the casual observer, or it can be so slight as to be virtually undetectable without special tests. Parents' concerns about their child's possible lazy eye should be investigated fully.

A "pseudo-lazy eye" is often seen in children who have especially marked folds of skin (epicanthic folds) above the near side of their eyes. These skin folds can give the appearance of a lazy eye by obscuring more of the white of the eye on the inner side. Specific tests (see below) will differentiate this effect from a true lazy eye. This characteristic is more commonly noticed in younger children before the development of definite strong facial features. Children who have a broad bridge to their nose, or who have an asymmetrical face for some reason, may also falsely appear to have a lazy eye. Again, special tests will differentiate such effects from real vision problems.

A **latent lazy eye** can become obvious when a child is ill with some intercurrent infection. Muscle control at this time is imperfect, and a lazy eye can be clearly seen. On recovery, the lazy eye will disappear, but it is prudent to consult an ophthalmologist to ensure that there is no permanent condition.

Lazy eye is not caused by anxiety, fear, or infectious disease, as some old wives' tales would have us believe.

INVESTIGATIONS

Tests for refractive errors: These will include tests for near-sightedness, far-sightedness, and astigmatism, with special reference to differences in the two eyes. (An astigmatism occurs when the lens of the eye is less than perfectly shaped, so that distorted images bounce off this ill-shaped refractive surface.)

Examination of light reflexes: Shining a light, from a pencil torch (for example), into the child's eye will show whether or not the reflection from the light occurs in the same position in each eye. If, for example, the light is reflected to the right of the pupil in one eye and over the pupil in the other, some degree of lazy eye is present.

The "cover test": This test involves covering one of the child's eyes with a hand, or card, while the child focuses on a distant object. On removal of the cover, the covered eye will be seen to move if a lazy eye is present. If there is no lazy eye, neither eye will move when the covering hand or card is removed. This test should be repeated two or three times in quick succession.

Orthoptic tests, with special equipment, to measure the angle of the lazy eye can be carried out once the presence of a definite lazy eye has been established.

Full examination by an ophthalmologist, with the eyes fully dilated, is necessary when causes other than simple refractive errors are suspected. Such an exam is vital to exclude serious eye disease.

MANAGEMENT

Correction of any refractive error is the first essential objective. An ophthalmologist will perform routine tests, appropriate to the age of the child, for farsightedness or near-sightedness, as well as for an astigmatism. Glasses are then prescribed to correct these errors. In many cases, glasses will result in an improvement of the lazy eye. It will be necessary to review constantly the strength of the visual correction. With growth, the refractive errors in a farsighted child can improve so much that the glasses can be discarded at a later date.

Occlusion of the good eye for one or two weeks at a time may be necessary to obtain good vision in the lazy eye. This treatment is often necessary if a degree of amblyopia has developed in the lazy eye.

Orthoptic exercises are also valuable in producing good binocular vision.

If the above treatments are not adequate, **surgery** under a general anesthetic can be necessary to correct the lazy eye. The muscles moving the eyes are lengthened, shortened, or repositioned according to the type and degree of the lazy eye.

Occasionally, **eyedrops** that cause accommodation of the lazy eye to decrease have been used with success to correct a small-angle lazy eye.

Other, more recent and experimental, treatments have been used to induce a temporary, partial **paralysis** of the eye muscles. This procedure allows time for binocular vision to become established.

THE FUTURE

Amblyopia can occur if a lazy eye remains undiagnosed and untreated for some time. Amblyopia becomes of great importance to the person if, at a late date, vision is lost in the normally seeing eye. Full vision can never be fully restored to an amblyopic eye.

Lice

INCIDENCE

There are three types of human lice—head lice, body lice, and "crabs" or pubic lice. The first two types are similar but merely affect different parts of the body—as evidenced by their names. Pubic lice are a different, quite distinct species.

Lice occur worldwide and are especially prominent in areas with low standards of hygiene. Head lice are the most commonly seen and will be the type described.

The incidence of head lice varies enormously from place to place and from time to time with no obvious explanation for these variations. During a head lice "epidemic," as many as 60% of children in schools can be affected at one time.

Infestation is most common in the 3- to 13-year-old age group—the incidence peaking among the 6- to 9-year-olds. Girls seem to be more commonly affected than boys. Strangely enough, hair length seems to have little bearing on whether lice are present or not. Both clean and dirty heads can be infested.

CAUSATION

Although head lice most frequently and most heavily infest the head, other hairy parts of the body can also be involved.

The insects live close to the roots of the hair, and feed on blood, which they suck from the underlying skin. The female lays around six to eight eggs ("nits") every 24 hours. These nits are stuck firmly to the shafts of hair and are initially found close to the scalp. As the hair grows, the nits will be found lower down the shaft away from the head. The eggs hatch within about ten days, and so the cycle is repeated, unless treatment to eradicate the lice—and the eggs—is given. The female louse lives for about a month, during which time she can lay around 240 eggs!

CHARACTERISTICS

There may be **no symptoms at all** in a child with a minimal number of head lice. The first clue as to an infestation may be the appearance of the characteristic white nits on the hair shafts.

Under conditions where there is a heavy infestation, the child's head may **itch**. This irritation is probably due to an allergic reaction to the presence of the lice and not to the movement of the insects. Any child who is continually scratching his or her head should be examined closely for the presence of lice. There are few other conditions in which there is such obvious irritation of the scalp alone. The most common places for lice to congregate are behind the ears and on the back of the head.

The constant itching of the scalp can cause the child to be a **restless sleeper.**

Excessive scratching of the scalp can cause an **infection** of the skin, giving rise to impetigo, which can cause a mild **fever** and, in severe cases, enlargement of the **glands in the neck.** Therefore, any child who has a mild fever and tender, swollen neck glands, but does not have a sore throat or other "cold" symptoms should have her or his head examined for head lice. If impetigo has occurred because of excessive scratching, antibiotic treatment will be required.

Head lice are transmitted through head-to-head contact, which is, of course, a very common event among small children, who frequently have their heads close together during play or during school activities. It is also thought that the lice can be passed on by sharing hair brushes and combs or by merely trying on the hat or other headgear of an infested playmate. Obviously, situations where there is overcrowding of children provide excellent conditions for head lice to infect a number of children.

MANAGEMENT

On discovery of an infestation in one child, the whole class—including the teaching staff—should have their heads examined for lice.

There are a number of preparations **(lotions and shampoos)** that effectively kill head lice. Lice rapidly become resistant to such treatments, so the type of preparation used in a location experiencing an infestation must be changed at fairly frequent intervals. Good liaison between health officials is necessary to preserve the efficacy of the preparations used.

The lotion or shampoo is applied to the child's head in the evening, allowed to dry naturally, and combed out the following morning. (The lotion is probably preferable to the shampoo.) One treatment should effectively kill all the lice, but the nits can remain stuck to the shafts of the hair and may need to be combed out with a fine-toothed nit comb. Success has also been achieved simply by **frequent combing** with a fine-toothed comb for a minimum of ten days. This approach must be followed conscientiously on a regular basis, while taking care not to make the child's head sore by overzealous combing.

There is no need to exclude the child from **school** once the treatment has been given. **Every member of the household** should have the lotion applied to his or her hair once one child in the family is found to be infested—even if no lice or nits are found on other children or parents. This will ensure that no minute, lurking louse will survive. (Care must be taken that the lotion does not splash into the child's eyes, as it will cause severe irritation. Also, care must be taken with the storage of the lotion—accidental ingestion by a toddler will require emergency treatment.)

PREVENTION

Rapid and adequate treatment of the whole family once an infested member is found is the best form of prevention once an initial child is infected.

Advise children not to borrow each other's hats, combs, etc.

Advise parents on adequate and frequent brushing, combing, and washing of children's hair.

Much emotion and upset can be caused at school when a child experiences an infestation with head lice, but it must be remembered that, once the lice are present in a class, they can just as easily pass to a beautifully clean head as to a less hygienic one!

Limp

INCIDENCE

The incidence of limping in children is not known, but this symptom is an important part of a variety of conditions. It is vital that any child who limps for any significant period of time should be fully investigated.

CAUSATION

The causes of a limp in children can range from the trivial, such as a blister or a plantar wart somewhere on the foot, to the serious, such as a septic arthritis or a tumor.

Signs and symptoms, as well as subsequent investigations and treatment, are related to the causative factor of the limp.

Conditions in the feet

Conditions such as warts, blisters, or a minor fracture following injury can cause a child to limp.

Blisters will need to be gently cleaned; no attempt should be made to burst the blister if the skin is still intact. A simple adhesive bandage and removal of the offending footwear is all the treatment that is necessary. (If the covering skin is removed from a blister—either accidentally or on purpose—exposing raw tissue, cellulitis can result. This inflammation of the connective tissues around the wound can spread alarmingly and affect the whole leg. Appropriate and rapid antibiotic treatment is necessary under these conditions.)

Plantar warts are a particularly common finding in the 11- to 16-year-old age group, and they can be sufficiently painful as to cause a limp at times. (This condition is addressed in the entry on warts.)

Fractures of the small bones of the foot can occur, sometimes after a seemingly minor injury. If the child describes either a crushing or a twisting injury, and is still in pain a day or two after the event, medical advice should be sought. An X-ray will confirm or exclude this cause for a limp.

Foreign bodies in the foot are a common hazard of childhood, especially if a child goes barefoot. Children will readily be able to point to the site of the implanted object. Removal will give relief and a return to a normal gait.

One of the **osteochondrites** (see the entry on Perthes disease) can affect the foot, causing a child to limp. Sever disease is an osteochondritis of the heel, while Kohler disease is a similar problem affecting one of the tiny bones of the foot. The typical picture of osteochondritis can be seen on X-ray. Immobilization in a cast for six to eight weeks may be necessary, although many milder cases will settle with a reduction in activity.

Juvenile chronic arthritis can first be manifested in the ankles. The child will complain of pain, and he or she can limp in an endeavor to relieve the discomfort. Such a limp can be one of the first signs of the poly- or pauciarticular types of juvenile arthritis (see the entry on arthritis).

Conditions in the hip

Perthes disease is another example of one of the osteochondrites—in this case, affecting the hip. A limp can be the only sign of this condition for some time.

A **slipped femoral epiphysis** can be another cause of a limp in an older child—usually in the early adolescent years. In this condition, the growing head of the femur gradually slips until it is in a nonaligned position relative to the pelvic bone. Occasionally, the condition can occur suddenly as a result of a twisting injury. Under these circumstances, the pain is acute and the child will be unable to move the affected leg. Boys are slightly more often affected than girls. Overweight children are thought to be more at risk from a slipped femoral epiphysis.

In addition to limping, the young person with a slipped femoral epiphysis is most likely to complain of pain in the knee—although the problem is in the hip. (Diseases of the hip often manifest themselves with pain referred to the knee joint. Therefore, any investigation of knee pain should include close examination of the hips.) On examination, there is swelling and limitation of the affected hip. X-ray examination will confirm the diagnosis. Operative procedures are necessary to realign the head of the femur in the pelvis.

"Irritable hip" (transient synovitis) is a relatively common condition that arises out of the blue and has no known specific causative factor. The child will limp, and the muscles around the hip joint will be in spasm. There may be an associated mild fever. Blood tests may also show a raised erythrocyte sedimentation rate (ESR). This condition usually settles adequately and quickly with a short period of bed rest.

Miscellaneous conditions

One of the most potentially disabling causes of a long-term limp is an undiagnosed (in babyhood) **congenital dislocation of the hip.** Fortunately, the hips of all babies are now routinely examined at birth and at subsequent progress checks. However, the possibility of this condition must always be remembered, particularly if the child has been born in a part of the world where such checks are not routinely performed.

Certain other—rare—conditions in which there is an **inequality in leg length** can cause a limp. Such conditions include a congenitally shortened bone in a leg, or scoliosis (a sideways twist in the spine that can be due to a variety of causes). An attack of poliomyelitis can cause a shortening of one leg—again, this cause is rare in developed countries, but it must be investigated as a possibility when a child has lived in a country where poliomyelitis is still endemic.

The possibility of a **tumor**—benign or malignant—in one of the leg bones must also be considered. Pain and swelling at the site of the tumor are the most usual manifestations of a growth, but a limp can also be one of the first signs in a younger child. Further investigations, followed by appropriate treatment, must be instigated rapidly if a tumor is suspected.

Finally, the possibility of **non-accidental injury** must always be considered when a child limps. Careful examination of the whole of the child's body must be undertaken, with follow-up X-rays if necessary, to exclude injuries for which there are no other apparent explanations.

Most limps in children are due to trivial and obvious causes, but important and treatable diseases can be missed if a long-term limp is ignored.

Measles

ALTERNATIVE NAME

Rubeola.

INCIDENCE

Hundreds of thousands of children every year suffered from this infection before the advent of immunization, and the incidence of the disease showed a marked biennial variation—every other year being a "bad" measles year.

Since the introduction of the measles vaccine in the 1960s, the incidence of the infection has fallen dramatically. The MMR (measles, mumps, and rubella) vaccine is now given routinely to all babies between the first and second years of life, and the annual number of cases of measles has dropped to several thousand.

Measles occurs most frequently in the 5- to 10-year-old age group, although in crowded urban conditions, many younger children also contract the infection. Measles is extremely rare in children under the age of 6 months, as antibodies from the mother protect the baby from the infection during those critical early months of life.

In developing countries, which have not benefited from the measles vaccine and in which childhood malnutrition is an ever-present problem, measles is a potent killer. As many as 25% of children in such nations die from this infection.

Most cases of measles today are comparatively mild, but complications can—and do—still occur. There are, regretfully, still a few deaths each year attributable to measles. Children who have other serious conditions, such as leukemia, are especially at risk.

CAUSATION

Measles is caused by a virus and is a highly infectious condition. Transmission occurs by droplet infection from the respiratory tract. The infection is usually passed on before the typical rash appears, and hence before a definite diagnosis of measles is made.

The incubation period is between 8 and 14 days.

CHARACTERISTICS

Measles begins in much the same way as does any common cold, with:

- a **runny nose,** associated with catarrhal symptoms;
- **sore, inflamed eyes** with marked photophobia (a dislike of light);
- a harsh, dry **cough;**
- a **fever** of varying degree;
- general **malaise;**
- and, in some cases, **convulsions** as a result of the high fever.

These are all very generalized symptoms, which can initially be attributed to any of a number of causes, such as the current upper respiratory tract infection that is "going around." Within two or three days, however, a very specific sign of measles can be noted in the child's mouth. Small white spots, which have been likened to grains of salt, appear on the insides of the cheeks opposite the back teeth. These are known as **Koplik spots** and only occur with an infection with the measles virus.

On the third or fourth day of the illness, the diagnosis becomes obvious with the appearance of the typical **rash,** which starts behind the ears and along the hairline before spreading rapidly to involve the whole body and limbs—the face and upper chest are usually the most affected parts of the body. The dusky red spots coalesce, giving rise to a blotchy appearance. The rash begins to fade after three or four days, often with some shedding of the surface skin.

With the appearance of the rash, a **high fever** can recur. This symptom will improve as the rash fades. In uncomplicated cases of measles, improvement is rapid following the disappearance of the rash, and the mildly affected child will be returned to full health within a week. Occasionally, the dry cough will persist for a week or two.

INVESTIGATIONS

Investigations are rarely, if ever, needed to make a diagnosis of measles, as the signs and symptoms are so definite once the rash has appeared. The virus can be isolated and grown from the secretions of the nose and throat as well as the urine of a sufferer.

COMPLICATIONS

The complications are potentially quite dangerous. For descriptive purposes, it is convenient to look at the problems that can develop in relationship to the body system involved.

Respiratory tract:

There is always an associated respiratory involvement with an attack of measles. The trachea (windpipe), larynx, and bronchi are all involved in this viral infection, as is evidenced by the sore throat and dry cough. **Secondary infection with bacteria** is a potential threat when the respiratory tissues are damaged by the measles virus. Bronchitis almost inevitably accompanies measles, and pneumonia is a common complication. Symptoms of further involvement of the respiratory tract include a return of fever and a worsening of the cough. Medical advice should always be sought if these symptoms should occur in a child who is getting over an attack of measles. Antibiotics, and perhaps hospital admission, will be necessary under these circumstances.

Central nervous system

Seizures can occur during the early stages of the infection. Medical advice should always be sought for a child who has had a seizure.

Encephalitis (inflammation of the brain) is the most serious complication of measles. The time at which signs and symptoms appear can vary, but most usually they occur around 7 to 10 days after the beginning of the illness. The child will become drowsy, suffer from seizures, and have a return of the fever. Specific neurological signs may also occur, such as weakening or paralysis of a limb. This serious state of affairs can show a steady slow improvement with no permanent after-effects; show a slow recovery, but leave the child with permanent neurological and/or intellectual damage; or show a steady deterioration resulting in a fatal outcome.

A rare form of encephalitis can occur some 5 to 10 years after an attack of measles. This is known as "subacute sclerosing panencephalitis" and is an extremely serious condition. The child first shows some loss of intellectual abilities, together with some instability of posture and difficulty in movement. This vicious condition progresses inexorably into paralysis and dementia and, finally, coma and death. This condition is thought to be due to a reactivation, by some unknown stimulus, of the measles virus, which has remained latent in the brain.

Eyes

The conjunctiva of the eye is involved to some degree in every case of measles, as is evidenced by the **photophobia** complained of by most children with measles.

Secondary bacterial infection can result in **irritation of the cornea.**

Ears

Otitis media used to be an almost invariable accompaniment to measles. Earache and high fever, along with the possible rupture of the eardrum and/or mastoiditis, added to the miseries of the child with measles. Fortunately, because of the apparently lower virulence of the measles virus today, as well as prompt antibiotic treatment, otitis media is now an unusual complication.

Gastrointestinal tract

The entire digestive system seems to be involved in the measles infection, ranging from soreness in the mouth to indigestion and abdominal pain. Lymph glands in the abdomen are also enlarged by the infectious process—yet one more uncomfortable and unpleasant aspect of this viral disease.

MANAGEMENT

Management will obviously differ for the child with complications and the child suffering from an uncomplicated attack of measles.

Uncomplicated measles

Adequate rest is necessary, in bed during the initial stages of the infection if symptoms are at all severe. When the child's temperature has settled and her/his energy is returning, quiet play in a warm room is permissible.

Adequate fluid intake is necessary to ensure that the child does not become dehydrated. High fever causes fluid loss through perspiration—and unwillingness to eat and drink also causes dehydration. Food should not be forced on the child, but plenty of drinks—of any kind—should be encouraged. **Acetaminophen** will help to lower temperature and can relieve headache and sore throat.

While a **darkened room** will not in any way improve the sore eyes so commonly associated with measles, the child will probably feel more comfortable in subdued light. Soothing eye-drops can also be prescribed.

Antibiotics have no part to play in an uncomplicated attack of measles. (These drugs are not active against viral infections.) However, if there is any suggestion of secondary bacterial infection anywhere in the body, antibiotics should be prescribed.

Complicated attack of measles

Antibiotics, usually penicillin, will be needed if respiratory or ear involvement occurs.

Neurological involvement will usually necessitate **hospitalization** for nursing, monitoring, and an adequate nutrition program.

Long-term management of the consequences of measles complications will depend on the amount of permanent damage. **Neurological and/or intellectual problems** will need **regular check-ups** for many months, as improvement can be maintained for some time after the initial infection has subsided. Special schooling should be arranged if necessary. **Hearing** should be checked a month or so after full recovery if the ears have been involved to any degree, as children can be left with varying degrees of deafness after measles.

Measles is an unpleasant disease with the potential for serious complications, and it should never be taken lightly. Fortunately, with the advent of immunization against the disease, the incidence has reduced dramatically. Nevertheless, measles does still occur and will continue to do so until at least 90% of children have benefited from the vaccine. Even mild cases can leave a child debilitated. It is wise to prevent the child from pursuing active pursuits for a week or two after recovery and to ensure that the convalescent child receives adequate rest and nutrition.

PREVENTION

Prevention is by **immunization.** The **MMR** vaccine is routinely administered when children are between 1 and 2 years old, and it is usually given once again before school entry. This vaccine should be given even if the child has been thought to have previously had an attack of naturally occurring measles. Age is no bar to receiving this vaccine if it has been missed at the usual time.

Contraindications to receiving the vaccine are the usual ones: if a child has an **acute feverish illness** at the time when the immunization is due, then the vaccine should be delayed until the child has recovered; also, children with any form of malignant disease and those receiving **immunosuppressant drugs** for any reason should not be vaccinated. If the child has a **severe reaction when eating eggs**—such as swelling of the mouth and throat or difficulty in breathing—she or he should not receive the vaccine; a child who merely dislikes eggs is not endangered by the vaccine.

THE FUTURE

An attack of measles confers immunity for life. Apart from the rare possibility of subacute sclerosing panencephalitis, or neurological or hearing damage from one of the complications, there are no adverse effects in later life from an attack of measles.

When immunization levels of children have reached the advised target, measles should be an infection of the past as is, for example, poliomyelitis today. Until that goal is reached, children will continue to suffer from measles.

Because measles is still a common, and much-feared, disease in developing countries, unimmunized individuals who travel to those areas are at risk of acquiring the infection.

Meningitis

INCIDENCE

Meningitis is caused both by viruses and by bacteria. The viruses that can cause meningitis are numerous; therefore, the exact incidence of cases of viral meningitis is difficult to classify.

Similarly, a number of bacteria can be responsible for bacterial meningitis (see below). Figures for meningococcal meningitis (caused by the bacterium *Neisseria meningitidis*) are well-documented, and the illness due to this cause can be seen to occur in peaks.

Meningitis due to bacteria is essentially an infection of childhood, and more than 80% of all cases affect children under the age of 15 years old. A high majority of these cases occur in children under the age of 5 years old.

CAUSATION

Among the **viruses** capable of causing meningitis are the viruses causing measles and mumps, the common Echo and Coxsackie viruses, Herpes simplex, and Epstein–Barr virus. A formidable list!

Bacteria that can cause meningitis are less numerous, but the number is still not inconsiderable. In the early days of life, meningitis is more often due to infection with certain types of *Streptococcus, E. coli,* and the *Hemophilus influenzae* type b bacterium. *Hemophilus influenzae* b (Hib) is the most common cause of meningitis in the 1- to 4-old age group.

CHARACTERISTICS

Whatever the infecting agent causing the illness, the characteristics (with a few exceptions) are similar.

Headache and/or **pain at the back of the neck** are among the most frequent early features. Associated with the pain at the back of the neck is a reluctance to bend the head forward. For example, the child cannot put his or her chin on his or her chest without exacerbating the pain in the back of the neck.

Nausea and **vomiting**—unassociated with abdominal pain—are also common features. The vomiting can be projectile in character.

Fever of varying degree usually accompanies these symptoms.

Photophobia (a dislike of light) can be marked, with the child turning away from the window and burying his or her face in the pillow.

Drowsiness and **irritability** on being disturbed can occur within a few hours.

Seizures can also occur.

With a specific type of meningitis—meningococcal meningitis—there is an associated **rash**. This rash is very specific, consisting of numerous, small, bruise-like spots all over the body, which do not fade on pressure. The rash is a sign of a serious infection that can be rapidly fatal—within hours—unless treatment is given.

In children younger than 2 years old, these characteristic signs are not so well marked. **Fever, vomiting,** and **pallor,** together with a **high-pitched cry** and **refusal of feedings,** can be the only initial signs of infection. Drowsiness and/or seizures are later serious signs in these younger children.

INVESTIGATIONS

A **lumbar puncture** to obtain cerebrospinal fluid must be performed in the hospital before treatment is started. (There is one major exception to this observation. If meningococcal meningitis is suspected—the distinctive rash being a strong diagnostic feature—immediate treatment with an antibiotic must be given without waiting for the lumbar puncture.) The cerebrospinal fluid thus obtained will appear cloudy in cases of meningitis. Laboratory examination will be able to determine the infecting agent.

Blood tests to determine the infecting agent are also useful.

MANAGEMENT

The child with meningitis can be seriously ill, and in many cases, hospitalization is necessary for treatment.

Antibiotic treatment is started immediately after the cerebrospinal fluid has been obtained by lumbar puncture. (The reason why treatment is not started before this investigation is done—except, of course, in the case of suspected meningococcal meningitis—is that treatment can confuse the laboratory diagnosis as to which infecting agent is present.) Ceftriaxone and/or chloramphenicol are the most usual antibiotics used, and it is usual to continue to give these drugs for at least ten days.

Fluids, which may initially given intravenously, can be necessary. The young child can become rapidly dehydrated if vomiting and fever are severe. Refusal to eat or drink also results in lack of fluid in the body.

Regular **monitoring** of the child's temperature, pulse, respiration, and level of consciousness is also necessary. If regular readings show any deterioration in the child's condition, immediate help can be given.

If seizures have occurred, or if the child is extremely restless, **anticonvulsant drugs** may be necessary for a short while.

Parents will need **emotional support** and perhaps also **physical help** (with other children or with traveling to the hospital, for example) during their child's serious illness.

With an uncomplicated attack of meningitis, recovery is complete with no permanent after-effects. Following discharge from the hospital, it is wise to allow the child a week or two of convalescence before she or he returns to the rough and tumble of the school day. Extra rest and a nutritious diet will help to restore general health following this serious illness.

COMPLICATIONS

Serious long-term complications can occur following a severe attack of meningitis. Probably the most common complication is **sensorineural deafness.** According to studies on the complications of meningitis, around 10% of children experience some degree of deafness following meningitis. All children should have their hearing tested a month or two after recovery from meningitis. Hearing aids and/or special schooling may be needed in the more severe cases. It is important that good liaison is maintained between health and education authorities involved with these children.

Epilepsy can be a late complication of meningitis. There does not appear to be any correlation between later epilepsy and the type of infecting organism. Children who have had seizures during the initial stages of their illness are most likely to develop later epilepsy. This complication reportedly affects around 5% of children following meningitis. Anticonvulsant drugs will be necessary to control seizures.

Mental retardation can be a sequel to meningitis. Parents or teachers may observe that the child's abilities have declined since the illness. Preschool children may lose skills previously learned, and these skills are only regained slowly. Regular developmental checks are necessary for the preschool child to determine the extent of the damage. These should be repeated regularly over succeeding months, as recovery can continue for some time after the acute stage of the illness is over. Again, special educational facilities may be required, with close liaison between health and education authorities.

Cerebral palsy, in which there are problems with control of the muscles of the body, can also occur after an attack of meningitis. Limbs can either become stiff and rigid with much difficulty in walking, or floppy and weak. Regular assessment by a pediatrician skilled in treating motor handicaps is vital. Physical therapy is also important to enable the child to make the most of his or her residual abilities. Speech problems may be arise as part of cerebral palsy, and help from a speech therapist is invaluable under these circumstances. Mental handicap and/or cerebral palsy are thought to affect 3 to 8% of children following an attack of meningitis.

PREVENTION

The meningitis caused by the *Hemophilus influenzae* type b bacterium—the most common type of meningitis seen in children between the ages of 1 and 4 years—is now preventable by **immunization.**

Immunization with this vaccine is part of the routine babyhood immunization schedule. Injections of the vaccine are given at the same time as the triple vaccine (against diphtheria, tetanus, and whooping cough) at 2, 4, 6, and 15 months of age. The vaccine affords protection for the child during the years when infection with this type of organism is at its height. Work is progressing on combining this vaccine with the triple vaccine.

There are **no contraindications** to a baby receiving this vaccine, apart from the usual ones of an acute illness (when the immunization should be postponed) or situations where there has been a severe reaction to a previous dose of vaccine. These reactions are virtually unknown. More than 20 million doses of this vaccine have been given, and no serious reactions have been reported. Minor reactions, such as redness and swelling around the injection site for a few hours, do occur, but they resolve rapidly.

There are no vaccines, or other preventive methods, against meningitis due to other infectious organisms.

During outbreaks of meningococcal meningitis in nurseries or schools, public health experts can determine the advisability of giving rifampin, or vaccine, to children who have had close contact with the individual suffering from this form of meningitis.

THE FUTURE

Following an attack of meningitis in childhood, there are no deleterious after-effects unless complications—as discussed above—have occurred. These, of course, can be severe, needing long-term specialized help.

Migraine

INCIDENCE

Migraine is rare in children younger than 2 years old. The incidence of this condition increases with age until, by school age, around 50 children in every 1,000 are thought to have suffered from an attack of migraine at one time or another.

Before puberty, the number of boys suffering from migraine is about twice the number of girls. At puberty, however, the number of male sufferers decreases and the number of females with migraines increases; among adults, incidence of attacks is greater for women than for men. Hormonal changes at around the time of puberty explain why the rates of incidence for males and females shift with age.

HISTORY

Socrates gave accounts of the classic signs of migraine some 25 centuries ago, so migraine is certainly not a new environmental disease! Lewis Carroll of *Alice in Wonderland* fame was known to suffer from severe attacks of migraine. The hallucinations of becoming smaller and smaller so graphically described in *Alice* are reminiscent of a certain specific late effect of migraine.

CAUSATION

Migraine is thought to be due to alterations in the reactions of the blood-vessels supplying the brain. In a migraine, there is a phase when these vessels constrict and become smaller, reducing the blood supply to particular parts of the brain. In a subsequent phase, the vessels dilate and the blood supply is increased. Different blood vessels can be affected at different times, a fact that probably accounts for the wide variety of symptoms seen in this condition.

These effects on the blood vessels are caused by a wide variety of stimuli, ranging from genetic susceptibility through reactions to certain foods and exercise to possible hormonal imbalances and reactions to viral infections.

Genetic predisposition: Ninety percent of children suffering from migraine have one or more members in their immediate family who also suffer from this condition.

Food: The foods most often implicated in the onset of an attack of migraine are **cheese** and **chocolate,** with **oranges** a close third. The two former foods contain a substance, tyramine, which is a powerful dilator of blood vessels. **Milk products, eggs,** and **gluten-containing foods** (i.e., wheat and wheat products) have at times also been considered to precipitate attacks of migraine. These foods may also precipitate other conditions (such as celiac disease, which results from an allergy to gluten), and the migraine may be but one symptom of a generalized food intolerance.

Other causes: Exercise, particularly if associated with competitive sports, may precipitate migraine in some children. In some athletic situations, it can be difficult to decide whether it is the exercise itself or the worry of the competition that causes the problem! (Under these circumstances, true migraine can easily be confused with so-called tension headaches.)

Sex hormones, androgens and estrogens, are probably responsible for the change in incidence of migraine seen at puberty. The extra androgens secreted by males around the time of puberty appear to reduce the tendency to migraine, while the increase in estrogen levels in females after puberty appear to increase the tendency. Changes in estrogen levels at various times in the menstrual cycle also influence the timing of attacks in some women.

A **viral infection** can precipitate an attack of migraine in a susceptible individual. In children, a migraine may be difficult to differentiate from the headache due to the infection itself. (With age and experience, the person suffering from migraine will become only too well aware of the difference!)

Given the number of possible causes, it is no wonder that migraine is so difficult to control.

CHARACTERISTICS

Migraine, for descriptive purposes, can be divided into a number of subtypes—all types are caused by changes in the blood vessels, but each has slightly differing symptoms.

Classical migraine has a very definite "aura" followed by a one-sided headache. This aura usually takes the form of visual manifestations, but specific smells have also been described. The visual aura can consist, for example, of blurring of the vision or flashes of light, perhaps in a zig-zag pattern. These visual effects are found in around 30% of children with migraine, and they can be very worrying to the child when they are first experienced. Headache usually follows on after the visual manifestations or the two symptoms can arise together.

Common migraine is less likely to be associated with an aura. The headache is also not so likely to be felt on one side of the head, but more as a generalized headache. Nausea and/or vomiting can accompany this type of migraine as well as general feelings of malaise.

Complicated migraine is said to occur when attacks of dizziness and/or periodic attacks of vomiting (known as "cyclical vomiting" or "abdominal migraine") occur. Under these circumstances, headache is not the most prominent feature of the attack. Children with this type of cyclical vomiting—which can also be accompanied by abdominal pain—frequently go on to develop the more usual forms of migraine in later life. It can be difficult to differentiate the attacks of dizziness from epilepsy, as the child can be so dizzy as to fall to the ground during a migraine.

Children with any form of migraine also appear to suffer from travel sickness more frequently than do other children—the figure quoted is about 40%.

INVESTIGATIONS

Before settling on a diagnosis of migraine, other physical causes for the headache must be excluded. Other serious conditions that could be the cause of the headache in children are brain tumors, continued bleeding into the brain following even a mild head injury, raised blood pressure, or undiagnosed hydrocephalus (an excess of fluid in specialized cavities of the brain).

As a brief guide, any child with a combination of the following symptoms should be checked to find the reason for the headaches:

- a headache that is **worse when waking** from sleep;
- a headache that **wakes him/her** from sleep;
- a headache that is **worse when coughing;**
- persistent **visual problems**—such as seeing colored lights or zig-zag lines for several days;
- a **behavior change** for no obvious reason;
- **neurological symptoms,** such as weakness of any part of the body; and
- **no family history** of migraine;

(Other less serious causes, such as sinusitis, should also be excluded before a diagnosis of migraine is made.)

Investigations under these circumstances include:

- checking **blood pressure,** after a careful history of the type and timing of the headaches has been taken;
- an **electroencephalogram,** especially if the child becomes drowsy or confused in association with the headaches.
- a **CT scan** if symptoms suggest that the headaches may be due to a serious and treatable cause.

If none of the pointers suggests a cause other than migraine, a few simple investigations will help to identify "triggering" factors, such as **stressful events.** Even such enjoyable events as birthday parties or theater visits, as well as competitive sports and exams, may trigger migraines. Parents should consult teachers regarding the child's progress in school—worries about difficulties in certain areas of schooling may cause headaches.

MANAGEMENT

Many of the migraine attacks suffered by both children and adults can be aborted if the individual **lies down** in a darkened, quiet room for an hour. This action is most frequently successful if it is taken before the attack is fully developed. Children who are used to attacks of migraine will know when an attack is imminent. Sympathetic parents and/or teachers (particularly those who suffer from migraine themselves) will encourage the child to lie down as soon as symptoms become obvious.

Analgesics, such as acetaminophen compounds, will also shorten an attack if taken early enough, particularly if combined with a period of rest.

Anti-emetic drugs, such as compazine, are useful if nausea and vomiting are a problem. If they are taken at the first warning signs of an attack, their effect can be greater.

Children with "cyclical vomiting" can benefit from regular treatment with one of the anti-emetic drugs. Such treatment can be especially helpful during a period of stress when attacks of vomiting and/or headache occur with monotonous regularity.

Drugs acting directly on the blood vessels are also available. Their use in children, however, is limited, both because of the type of migraine commonly suffered by children and because of the side effects of these drugs. Only in intractable migraine, and then under strict medical supervision, are these drugs used to treat children.

Biofeedback techniques have been tried with some children, with varying degrees of success. Here, skin resistance and blood flow are measured and then techniques to alter these measurements are used.

Elimination diets can be tried for children whose migraines have not been relieved by other methods if a food component is thought to play a part in triggering the attacks.

Commonsense handling of the attacks by all adults involved with the child is important. Too much emphasis on the migraine will cause concern, which can trigger additional attacks. The difficult balancing act between sympathetic understanding and encouragement is an art to be learned by all parents of children who suffer from migraine.

PREVENTION

Avoiding foods that are known to bring on an attack is an obvious way to prevent migraine.

Stressful situations can to a certain extent be controlled as the child matures and becomes more in control of both his/her environment and his/her reactions to stress. If a child has learning difficulties, specialized instruction can do much to relieve the stress of repeated failure.

THE FUTURE

Migraine fortunately tends to decrease both in frequency and severity with age, but in some cases, such relief may not be found until early middle age. The teenage years and the 20s and 30s can be trying, but experience will show the individual how best to avoid or abort attacks.

Mononucleosis

ALTERNATIVE NAMES

Infectious mononucleosis; "kissing disease."

INCIDENCE

Mononucleosis is a disease that usually affects older children and young adolescents. However, younger children are by no means immune to the condition, although children under the age of 3 years rarely suffer from the disease.

Overcrowding and poor hygiene are factors in the spread of the infection, which is transmitted by close physical contact. The virus is harbored in the throat and salivary glands—often for many months after recovery from the original infection. (This fact is the reason why mononucleosis is popularly known as the "kissing disease"; mouth-to-mouth contact is a likely means of spreading the disease during the adolescent years.) Epidemics can occur in schools and residential homes.

There is no particular time of the year when mononucleosis is more common; cases occur throughout the seasons.

The infection is found worldwide and affects both sexes.

HISTORY

The incidence of mononucleosis appears to have changed since the early twentieth century, when younger children were the most frequent sufferers, and epidemics among that age group were described.

CAUSATION

Mononucleosis is caused by a virus of the Herpes group—the Epstein–Barr virus. The incubation period is thought to be between 5 and 10 days. Because the virus remains in the throat and salivary glands, infection can spread to a second person up to 12 weeks after first individual experienced the initial attack.

CHARACTERISTICS

Mononucleosis can be notoriously difficult to diagnose clinically because there are a number of different ways in which the infection can manifest itself and because signs and symptoms of the disease are sometimes very similar to those of other infectious conditions, such as tonsillitis or influenza.

Characteristically, however, mononucleosis begins with **tiredness** and a general feeling of **malaise** with **headache, muscular pain, sore throat,** and **fever**—all of which are very general signs of any infectious illness. In mononucleosis, however, many of the **glands in the neck** become swollen. Swelling of the **glands in the armpit and groin** soon follow.

Occasionally in children, there is a transient **rash** at the onset of the disease. (If ampicillin, an antibiotic commonly used to control infections, is given to a child who has mononucleosis, a severe rash can be the result.)

The **tonsils** appear red and swollen (a very similar picture to that seen in an attack of tonsillitis). In severe cases, swallowing can be difficult for the youngster.

On close examination of the mouth, tiny hemorrhages are seen on the **palate** in the early stages of the infection. This sign is specific to mononucleosis, and it can help to make the diagnosis clear if seen early enough in the infection.

The **spleen** is enlarged and often tender to touch. Also, the **liver** is often enlarged, and **jaundice** may be a feature.

INVESTIGATIONS

Blood tests show a specific feature, an excess in the number of a particular type of white cells. A specific test on the blood, the Paul–Bunnell reaction, confirms the diagnosis of mononucleosis, but it is only positive in 60% of cases. There is a similar rapid slide test, the "monospot" test, which can be performed quickly in some clinics without the need to wait for laboratory results. Both these tests can be negative in the early stages of the disease—yet another complication—but they will be positive if repeated a week later.

Other **specific laboratory tests** done on a blood sample will show changes that will help with the diagnosis.

MANAGEMENT

There is no specific treatment for an attack of mononucleosis. Acyclovir—a useful drug against some viral infections under certain conditions—is of no value against infection with the Epstein–Barr virus.

Rest (not necessarily in bed), with **adequate fluids** and a **light diet,** together with analgesics to relieve the pain of the sore throat and headache and plenty of sympathy are the only treatments available.

A **throat swab** should be taken if the tonsillar involvement is severe and the glands in the neck are tender as well as swollen. At times, a secondary infection with *Streptococcus* bacteria can add to the patient's miseries. Under these circumstances, treatment with penicillin is indicated.

Most children will completely recover from an attack of mononucleosis within three weeks, although the feelings of malaise, mild fever, and lack of appetite can drag on for weeks or months in some cases. Under these conditions, it is wise to for a chest X-ray to be taken to exclude any further infection in the lungs.

Older children may have difficulties at school if they succumb to an attack of mononucleosis. There is no doubt that the child will not be able to give of his or her best if he or she has only recently recovered from mononucleosis. Most educational authorities recognize this fact and make the appropriate allowances.

COMPLICATIONS

Secondary bacterial infection can occur in throat or lungs, as mentioned above, and must be treated with the appropriate antibiotic.

Liver involvement, giving rise to jaundice, rarely occurs in children. If it does, recovery will be complete and rapid.

Occasionally, there can be a **relapse,** with symptoms similar to the original attack after a few weeks. Symptoms will resolve spontaneously with a few days rest.

PREVENTION

Sensible precautions, such as good hygiene, avoidance of overcrowding, and minimal close contact with the individual with the infection, are all that can be done by way of preventative measures.

THE FUTURE

There are no long-term after-effects from mononucleosis.

Mumps

ALTERNATIVE NAME

Epidemic parotitis.

INCIDENCE

Children of both sexes between the ages of 5 and 15 years are the usual sufferers from an attack of mumps. It is rare in children younger than 5 years old.

HISTORY

The word "mump" is an Old English term meaning "mope"—a good description of someone with the uncomfortably swollen face of mumps!

CAUSATION

Mumps is an infectious disease of the salivary glands caused by a specific virus. The parotid salivary glands situated on each side of the face below and in front of the ears are the glands most commonly—and obviously—affected. The other salivary glands, beneath the chin and tongue, are also frequently affected.

The condition is spread by droplet infection from the breath of a person with mumps. Children are infectious for several days before the obvious signs of mumps appear. The incubation period of the disease is 14 to 21 days. The infection can be passed on for several days after the swelling of the glands becomes apparent.

Immunity to the virus is lifelong following an attack of mumps.

CHARACTERISTICS

As with many of the infectious "childhood" fevers, mumps can begin with the very general symptoms of **headache, fever, loss of appetite,** and a general feeling of ill-health. Within two or three days, however, the diagnosis will become obvious when **pain and swelling in the parotid glands** (and possibly the other salivary glands as well) occur. Occasionally, this swelling can be the first sign of the condition, the usual prodromal symptoms being absent. Either one or both of the parotid glands can be involved. The swellings may be small, or they can be very large and extremely painful and tender. Sometimes the swelling on one side of the face will disappear, only to be replaced by swelling in the opposite parotid gland. Regardless of the variation of symptoms that occurs, a person with mumps gains immunity against future attacks of the infection.

Eating or drinking can cause extreme pain in the affected glands at the height of the infection.

A **dry mouth** is also a common complaint with an attack of mumps, as the amounts of saliva secreted by the affected salivary glands fall well below normal levels.

INVESTIGATIONS

Laboratory tests from saliva swabs can give positive proof of infection with the mumps virus. However, such tests are rarely done, as diagnosis can usually be made on clinical grounds.

MANAGEMENT

There is no specific treatment for an attack of mumps.

Analgesics are necessary to control the pain in cases where the parotid glands are swollen and tender. It is a good idea to give a painkiller about half an hour before a meal in order to reduce the pain caused by attempted salivary secretion from the inflamed gland. These useful drugs—such as acetaminophen—will also help to lower fever, and so make the young patient feel more comfortable.

A **suitable diet** is helpful during the height of an attack of mumps. When the swelling is extreme, it may be necessary to restrict the child to fluids only. After swelling diminishes, **easily swallowed foods** such as soups, jello, ice cream, and liquidized foods are best.

Children will need to **remain out of school** until the worst of the swelling of the parotid glands has subsided, for they will remain highly infectious until four or five days after the appearance of the swelling. After that time, schooling can be resumed with no risk to children in contact with the sufferer, always provided, of course, that the child is feeling completely well again.

COMPLICATIONS

Complications can be an important factor in an otherwise mild infectious disease.

Meningitis can be caused by the mumps virus. Occasionally, signs and symptoms of meningitis can be the first clue that a child is suffering from infection with the mumps virus. At other times, the meningitis occurs along with the swelling in the parotid glands or after the worst of the swelling has subsided—as long as ten days later. Signs of meningitis are **fever** (or a return of fever once the fever due to the original infection has subsided), **headache,** a **stiff neck,** and, at times, a **sore throat.**

Hospital admission is usually necessary for a child with mumps meningitis. A lumbar puncture will confirm the diagnosis following laboratory examination of the cerebrospinal fluid thus obtained. As a side effect, the lumbar puncture can bring rapid relief of headache.

There is no specific treatment for mumps meningitis, apart from good nursing care. (Antibiotics are of no value, as they are inactive against viral infections.) Recovery is usually complete, but, sadly, permanent brain damage can result from severe mumps meningitis.

Unilateral deafness can also be a residual handicap following mumps. Children who have had a severe attack of mumps and in whom deafness is suspected by the parents, or any child who has suffered from meningitis due to this infection, should receive a hearing test a few weeks following recovery from the infection. It can be all too easy to miss this complication, particularly in younger children.

Orchitis is another possible complication of an attack of mumps, but it is rare before puberty. In this condition, one or both testes become acutely painful, red, and swollen. Treatment is again nonspecific. Support of the inflamed testes with appropriate firm bandages can be helpful, as can ice-bags applied to the hot, swollen organ. Frequent painkillers can also be necessary. Sterility is by no means the inevitable outcome of mumps orchitis, as was once thought. Parents of young boys should be firmly reassured on this point.

Pancreatitis, in which the pancreas becomes involved in the general infection, is a rare complication, but it can be the cause of acute abdominal pain during an attack of mumps. There is usually no permanent damage to the pancreas, but, in very rare cases, diabetes can subsequently occur.

PREVENTION

Immunization against mumps is possible with the **MMR** (measles, mumps, and rubella) vaccine, which is now routinely given to children when they are around 15 months old. Only one injection is necessary to ensure immunity to mumps. There is a risk of other members of the family acquiring any of the three infections from a younger, recently immunized, member.

Immunization should be postponed if the child due to receive the injection has any acute illness. Also, children receiving immunotherapy for other serious illnesses should not be given this immunization. The only other contraindication to receiving the vaccine is a proven allergy to the antibiotic neomycin or a serious reaction to eating eggs (egg products are used in the making of the vaccine). Mere dislike of eggs is no reason for omitting the vaccine.

The immunization can be given to children of any age.

THE FUTURE

With the advent of immunization against mumps, this infection should eventually be eliminated. Mumps vaccine has been given to children for more than 20 years, and there has been a dramatic drop in the number of reported infections and complications due to mumps.

Otitis Media

ALTERNATIVE NAME

Middle ear infection.

INCIDENCE

The true incidence of otitis media is not known, but any pediatrician will see a number of children with this condition every week.

Boys and girls of all races are equally affected.

The incidence of this infection is higher in cool, temperate climates during the winter months—when upper respiratory infections are at their height. Throat infections and/or tonsillitis frequently precede, or coexist with, acute otitis media.

HISTORY

Before treatment of otitis media with antibiotics became routine in the 1950s, mastoiditis (infection in the bony mastoid process) was a relatively common condition. The mastoid process is situated behind and below the ears. This bony process readily becomes infected following a severe untreated case of otitis media. This infection was a serious consequence of otitis media, with meningitis as another possible sequel. Operation on the mastoid process was necessary to remove and drain the infected bone. Older people still show the scars of this procedure, along with the deafness that was often also the residual result.

CAUSATION

The infecting organisms in otitis media can be either bacteria or viruses. Around half of the infections are probably due to a viral cause, but secondary bacterial infection is common.

CHARACTERISTICS

Pain in the ear is the outstanding feature of acute otitis media. Even very young children accurately pinpoint the source of their pain when they clasp a hand over the affected ear, or rub it along the blanket or sheet. This pain can be one of the reasons for frequent waking in the night.

Fever, sometimes high, is a frequent accompaniment of an acute ear infection.

Associated **coughs** and **colds** are also common. These are due to the easy spread of infection up the eustachian tube into the middle ear.

On examination with an otoscope in the early stages of the infection, the **eardrum** appears **reddened** and covered with **dilated blood vessels.** Later, the delicate tissue of the drum will appear unusually **dull** and **congested** and bulge into the external auditory meatus. Ultimately, if no treatment has been available, the eardrum can **rupture** into the external auditory meatus. When that occurs, the pain will ease (because of the release of pressure) and a discharge of blood and pus will flow from the affected ear. Otitis media should never be allowed to reach this stage. Deafness can be a permanent late effect of rupture of the eardrum. The scar tissue that replaces the hole in the drum reduces the elasticity, and hence the adequate function, of this vital part of the hearing mechanism.

MANAGEMENT

Earache in children must always be regarded as an emergency, and medical help should be sought as soon as possible. Early treatment with **antibiotics** is essential if permanent damage to hearing is to be avoided. The pain from most attacks of otitis media usually clears up within 24 hours of starting treatment, but it is important that the full course of a prescribed antibiotic should be finished, in order to eradicate fully the infection.

If the pain does not subside after a couple of days treatment with a specific antibiotic, it will be necessary to get a different one prescribed.

Analgesics, such as acetaminophen, should be given in the early painful stages of otitis media; these drugs will also help to reduce fever.

A **hearing test** should ideally be performed approximately three months after a severe attack of otitis media to ensure that the infection has not left the child with the complication of secretory otitis media.

COMPLICATIONS

Secretory otitis media ("glue ear")

Causation: The cause of secretory otitis media, which can sometimes follow acute otitis media, is unclear. It is perhaps due to lack of proper drainage of secretions via the eustachian tube. This tiny tube can easily become blocked by mucus, or by swelling of the surrounding tissues, and the blockage can cause a build-up of sticky fluid in the middle ear. In turn, this fluid restricts the movement of the eardrum and so prevents sound waves from traveling clearly to the nerves of hearing.

Characteristics: Secretory otitis media can be difficult to pinpoint. A child's hearing can be perfectly normal for several days, but for the next week or two, it can be very restricted due to a further build-up of fluid. The first signs of hearing loss can be **lack of attention** in school, or the tendency to **turn up the volume** on the television to an extraordinarily high level. **Behavioral problems,** too, can have their basis in a hearing loss. The unfortunate child cannot hear clearly what is being said in class, becomes frustrated, and therefore "switches off" altogether or reacts in a generally antisocial manner. In younger children with this problem, the proper development of speech can be hindered.

Investigations: If secretory otitis media is suspected, an ear, nose, and throat surgeon should examine the child's eardrums and perform specialized hearing tests such as impedance audiometry.

Management: This can be difficult, but includes trying the following.

Decongestant nose drops and **antihistamine drugs** have both been prescribed over the years, but regretfully both can have less than satisfactory results.

Another possible procedure is **myringotomy,** in which the eardrum is pierced, under a general anesthetic, and the sticky fluid is withdrawn. A tiny ventilation tube is then placed in the eardrum to allow air into the cavity of the middle ear and so prevent the repeated build-up of fluid. Tubes rarely, if ever, need to be removed from their position in the eardrum. They fall out spontaneously, usually within a year to 18 months of their insertion. (The tubes are so tiny that parents are usually quite unaware that they have been extruded. It is not until the ears are again examined with an otoscope that the tubes are found to be missing.) There has been much controversy over the years regarding the vexed question of whether or not children with tubes in their ears should be allowed to swim. It is unlikely that any harm will come to the middle ear if small amounts of water make their way into the external auditory canal. It is wise, however, to ban such activities as diving under water if a child has tubes in his or her ears.

Hearing aids, as a temporary measure, are gaining in popularity for the treatment of secretory otitis media (see the entry on deafness).

THE FUTURE

If treatment for an acute attack of otitis media is prompt and adequate, and if secretory otitis media is diagnosed quickly, most children will have normal hearing and few attacks of earache by the time they are 7 or 8 years old.

Perthes Disease

ALTERNATIVE NAMES

Legg–Calvé–Perthes disease; coxa magna; osteochondritis.

INCIDENCE

Exact figures for this condition are not known, but it is thought that around 1 in every 2,000 children is affected. Perthes disease occurs in children between the ages of 2 and 12 years old, and most cases are seen in children between the ages of 4 and 8 years old. Boys are approximately four times more frequently affected than are girls. A few children with Perthes disease have the condition in both hips.

While there is no discernible genetic cause, brothers and sisters of individuals with Perthes disease have a slightly higher chance of having the condition than does the general child population.

CAUSATION

Exactly why this condition should occur is uncertain. A temporary diminution in the blood-supply to the head of the femur, or thigh bone, (the "ball" of the "ball-and-socket" hip joint) is the most probable cause. This blood problem, together with the compression exerted on this weight-bearing joint, are thought to be the two etiological factors.

In addition to bony changes, there is swelling of the surrounding soft tissues. These two factors eventually lead to destruction of the normal anatomy of the joint. It is these changes that give rise to the typical characteristics of the condition.

CHARACTERISTICS

Any child with a **limp** that lasts for longer than a few days should be investigated thoroughly, as a limp, associated with an unusual, lurching gait, can be one of the first signs of Perthes disease—evident even before the child complains of pain.

When it does occur, **pain** can be felt either in the affected joint itself or referred down the thigh into the knee. This pain can vary in intensity from day to day, although it is usually consistently worse after exercise.

158

(Strangely enough, the degree of pain seems to bear little relationship to the changes seen on X-ray. Therefore, it is important that even a mild degree of pain should be thoroughly investigated.)

On examination of the leg, there is found to be a **limitation of movement** of the hip, which is caused by muscle spasm in an effort to protect the joint. The child will also actively dislike attempts to move the hip joint.

There are rarely any severe constitutional symptoms with Perthes disease.

INVESTIGATIONS

X-ray of the affected joint will allow a definitive diagnosis, as the changes seen are quite typical of the condition. The space between the head of the thigh bone and the pelvis is wider than usual, due to the swelling of the surrounding soft tissues. With advanced disease, the usual smooth surface of the "ball" of the hip joint appears irregular and it may contain cysts. It is when the actual growing part of the bone is affected that permanent damage—such as a shortening of the affected leg—can occur.

Following treatment, regular X-rays, at about three-month intervals, are necessary to review progress. The hip joint will eventually heal and recalcify. The degree of residual disability will depend on the amount of bony destruction that has occurred during the active stages of the disease.

MANAGEMENT

In the initial stages of the disease, **bed rest with the affected leg in traction** is necessary. The leg is held in an immobile raised position to allow the hip to heal without the stresses and strains on the joint that inevitably occur when the child is walking or running. **Physical therapy** is vital during this stage to ensure that the muscles in the legs do not become weak during this period of inactivity.

Analgesics of appropriate type and dosage should be given if pain is severe.

Children of school age with Perthes disease will need help with their **education** because of their unavoidable absences from school during treatment. Contact with the child's school can often be arranged, with appropriate work and activities sent to the child. Such assignments will obviate much of the boredom and frustration of enforced inactivity as well as keeping the young patient in touch with events at school.

Depending on the stage of the disease as seen on X-ray, the hip can eventually be immobilized in a special type of **splint** with the leg held outward and rotated inward. This position is an incredibly awkward one, but children quickly adapt to it and become quite mobile. With some rearrangement in the classroom and a sympathetic teacher, the child can once again attend school. This form of immobilization will need to be continued for several months.

Time off from school will be necessary for continuing **physical therapy** to ensure that unused muscles do not become weak. Again, sympathetic understanding on the part of the child's teacher is vital.

Emotional support for both parents and child will be necessary during the long period of immobilization of the affected leg. Encouragement from the orthopedic consultant, pediatrician, and school can do much to help.

THE FUTURE

Depending on the severity of the Perthes disease, there may be, in a few children, some **shortening** of the leg on the affected side. This consequence will only occur if the actual growing part of the bone has been affected. Usually, little effect is noticed even if this has occurred.

Adults who had Perthes disease in childhood may develop **osteoarthritis** in the affected hip.

RELATED CONDITIONS

Osteochondritis is not confined to the hip joint. Other joints, and particular parts of bones, can also be affected. The disease process is exactly the same as in Perthes disease. These osteochondrites are given different names, which indicate the bone affected.

Osgood–Schlatter disease

This disease is osteochondritis of the tibial tubercle—the small bony projection in the shin bone just below the knee.

Osgood–Schlatter disease usually occurs in boys around the time of puberty. There is a painful swelling in this position on the leg, causing the boy to walk with a limp. X-ray changes are similar to those seen in Perthes disease.

Treatment is by immobilization in a cast for six to eight weeks, or temporary restriction of vigorous activity in mild cases. Following such treatment, a gradual return to full activity, over the succeeding two months or so, is advisable. The help of a physical therapist is valuable in strengthening muscles weakened by inactivity.

Sever disease

In this condition, it is the heel bone that is involved. X-ray changes resemble those seen in other types of osteochondritis, and the child will find walking painful. Once again, this condition occurs more commonly in adolescence. A walking cast may be necessary for around six weeks to relieve pain, although fitting a raised heel to the shoe can sometimes give sufficient relief.

Kohler disease

A small bone in the foot is the site of the osteochondritis in Kohler disease. Boys between the ages of 3 and 8 years are most commonly affected. A limp, with local pain and tenderness in the foot, are the symptoms of Kohler disease. Walking tends to aggravate the pain.

A six to eight week period of immobilization in a walking cast will promote recovery.

THE FUTURE

All the above conditions heal readily and leave no permanent after-effects.

Pinworm

INCIDENCE

Pinworms are common throughout the world and are—surprisingly—especially common in countries with a colder climate. The age group most often affected are boys and girls between the ages of 5 and 9 years old. (Research from the late 1980s suggests that there is a further peak in incidence between the ages of 30 and 49 years old. One possible explanation from this finding is that persons in this age group are most likely to live with 5- to 9-year-olds and so are infected along with their children.)

Infestation occurs more commonly in urban areas.

CAUSATION

Infestation with pinworms is passed on from child to child by hand contact, or through contact with soiled underclothes or bed linens. The tiny eggs of the pinworm are laid, in many thousands, around the child's anus. These eggs can then be transferred from the anus to fingers to the mouth. The eggs hatch on their way through the intestine. The adult worms then mate, and the female again lays further thousands of eggs, repeating the cycle. The eggs can survive in dust, at room temperature, for up to 2 or 3 weeks.

Domestic animals play no part in the dissemination of pinworms, making the mode of spread different from that of other worms.

CHARACTERISTICS

Over the years, pinworms have been blamed for causing many symptoms in children—nail-biting, convulsions, and hyperactivity, to mention just a few. None of these conditions are due to pinworms.

The presence of worms can cause **irritation around the anus,** as well as **sleep disturbances.** Some authorities also think that the worm can cause **bed wetting.** In girls, **irritation around the vulval area** can result from infestation with pinworms.

Parents can also, at times, be alarmed to see worms in their child's stools. However, worms are not seen as frequently as might be expected, because of the smallness of the worms, which are only around 10 millimeters long.

INVESTIGATIONS

The best method to determine whether or not a child is infested with pin-worms is for a medical practitioner to wrap a piece of tape (sticky side out) around a test-tube or spatula and apply this to the child's anus. The tape is then transferred to a microscope slide. The eggs, if present, can readily be seen under the microscope. (The child should not have bathed or had a bowel movement before this test is performed.) It may be neces-sary to repeat this investigation for three consecutive days, as the worms do not necessarily pass through the intestine in a regular manner.

MANAGEMENT

There are a number of **drugs** that will effectively eliminate pinworms. Usually, only one dose is needed. It is advisable that all members of the family should be treated, because of the many thousands of eggs that can be present in the bed linens and the general household dust.

Hygiene, especially personal cleanliness, is vital to control infesta-tions with pinworms. Children should be taught the importance of **wash-ing their hands** before meals and after using the toilet. **Fingernails** should be cut short to reduce the possibility of the eggs remaining under the nails. Frequent changes of underwear and bed linens are also impor-tant in the control of infestation with pinworms.

Parents will need **reassurance** that they are not alone in having pin-worms as visitors to their family and that their child will not suffer per-manent harm.

COMPLICATIONS

Very occasionally, there may be such a heavy infestation of pinworms in the bowel that the child may complain of **abdominal pain.** This pain can be cured by the appropriate treatment to eliminate the worms. (Pinworms have been found in the lumen of the appendix following removal of this organ, but it is not thought that their presence has any bearing on the onset of the appendicitis.)

PREVENTION

Prevention is limited to good personal hygiene and prompt and adequate treatment of the whole family if an infestation is found to be present.

Pityriasis

INCIDENCE

Pityriasis rosea is an uncommon condition, but it can give rise to much concern because of the extensive rash that is the main feature of the disease. Older children—over the age of 10 years—are the most usual sufferers. Pityriasis rosea is frequently found during adolescence.

All races are equally affected, as are both sexes. Some authorities say that one attack of pityriasis confers immunity for life, but this opinion is by no means necessarily valid.

Pityriasis alba is a similar condition, but it is rarely seen.

HISTORY

Pityriasis has been recognized for centuries. Pityriasis is a word derived from the Greek meaning "bran," a word that aptly describes the flaky scales on the skin characteristic of the condition.

CAUSATION

The exact cause of pityriasis is not clearly known. Various theories have had their vogue, ranging from a fungal infection through an allergic manifestation to a viral origin. It is now thought that the latter is the true cause, although no specific virus has so far been isolated.

Cases of pityriasis tend to occur in clusters. This fact adds extra force to the infectious theory.

CHARACTERISTICS

Characteristically, pityriasis begins with one lesion on the skin, known as the **herald patch.** It is a single, round eruption that can occur anywhere on the body, but it most usually appears on the chest, back, or upper limbs. This patch can be up to ten centimeters in diameter, and it has a typical scaly appearance, often with a patch of clear skin in the center.

Within a week or two, an **extensive rash** develops all over the body. Fortunately, hands, feet, and face are usually spared, although the rash does occasionally extend to these exposed sites of the body. More of the rash tends to appear every two or three days for around a week. The rapidness with which the rash spreads can be quite alarming, particularly for a self-conscious adolescent. The rash **may be itchy,** but that is not always the case.

The rash will gradually disappear, but it will be between three and eight weeks before the skin is finally completely clear—again a source of much distress. As with the herald patch, the lesions will clear initially in the centers, leaving a ruff of bran-like scales around the edges of the spots. Eventually the rash will disappear completely, leaving no residual trace of the once extensive eruption.

Very occasionally, there may be a mild fever and a general feeling of ill-health before the rash becomes apparent, but this finding is unusual.

MANAGEMENT

There is little that can be done to speed the cure of this trivial, but nevertheless distressing, condition. If irritation is a problem, a **steroid cream** can be helpful, or an **antihistamine** may be given at night.

Reassurance that, within a few weeks, the rash will completely disappear is important. As mentioned previously, recurrence is rare, but it can occur—often many years later.

There is no need for children with pityriasis to stay away from **school,** although it is important that teachers—and other parents!—are reassured that the extensive rash is not infectious.

THE FUTURE

There are no adverse effects following an attack of pityriasis rosea.

Psoriasis

INCIDENCE

Psoriasis is known worldwide and affects people of all races. It is usually thought of as a disease of adult life, but it can, in fact, occur in the youngest of children. A particular type of diaper rash, which is very resistant to the usual forms of treatment, may be due to psoriasis.

Both sexes can be affected, although more girls than boys have psoriasis. There is often a strong family history of the condition.

HISTORY

It is possible that some of the leprous lesions described in antiquity may have been due to psoriasis.

CAUSATION

Psoriasis is considered to be a dominantly inherited disorder. If one parent has the condition, one out of four of their children will stand a chance of inheriting the disease. (Regretfully, there is no way of predicting if an individual child will be affected. If, for example, the first child in the family has psoriasis, that does not mean that the next three children will be free of the condition. The chances are one in four for each successive child.)

Faults in immunological function and also hormonal imbalance are thought to be implicated in psoriasis.

The onset of psoriasis frequently occurs following a bout of infection or any other form of stress, such as an accident or a bereavement.

CHARACTERISTICS

In children, psoriasis usually begins in a slightly different form from the lesions seen in the adult form of the disease. The **rash** consists of small patches, or "drops" (the name **guttate psoriasis**—*gutta* meaning "a drop" in Latin—is applied to these early lesions). The rash can appear anywhere on the body, including the face.

As the child matures, the rash changes its characteristics to resemble the more adult form. This rash consists of larger **plaques** with a **white,** scaly surface, mainly on the knees, elbows, and scalp. In children, the rash of psoriasis is often preceded by an **upper respiratory tract infection** with the *Streptococcus* bacteria.

When psoriasis affects armpits, groin, or the diaper area in babies, the scaliness is less evident and the rash is red and angry-looking. Typically, the edges of the rash of psoriasis have a well-defined margin. The rash does not itch.

Psoriasis is a condition that fluctuates in severity throughout life. Periods of stress or infection often increase the amount of rash seen. Psoriasis is **not an infectious condition,** a fact that should be explained fully to parents and teachers as well as to the children themselves.

MANAGEMENT

Psoriasis is a skin condition for which there is no complete cure. However, much improvement can be gained by the various forms of treatment available. It is important that both child and parent should understand that there is no cure, so that the disappointment is not too great when the rash recurs. **Encouragement** to persevere with treatment and **emotional support** are vital as the child matures and learns to live with the inherited skin condition.

Sunlight usually has a beneficial effect on psoriasis. Therefore, in the summertime, children and adolescents should be encouraged to expose arms and legs affected by a psoriasis rash rather than covering up the scaly lesions in an attempt to hide them from other people.

Preparations in the form of ointments or pastes—based on tar and salicylic acid—are the most suitable for use in children. There are a wide range of these preparations, and trial and error will determine which one is of the most benefit to each individual child.

Weak **steroid preparations** are also useful. These should be used for a short time only, because of the possible side effects that can occur with these drugs. Unfortunately, there is often a relapse once these preparations are no longer applied.

If the child has an upper respiratory tract infection at a time when the rash is at its worst, a course of **penicillin** will often clear the rash as well as curing the respiratory tract infection.

Long-term follow-up of children with this unpleasant condition is important.

Children with psoriasis can suffer from taunts at school. Such situations will require sympathetic handling by teachers, who should be informed of the noninfectious—and recurrent—nature of the condition.

Certain **careers** will be inadvisable for individuals with psoriasis. They should be advised against considering careers in chemistry, in the beauty industry, or in certain artistic activities.

COMPLICATIONS

Psoriasis is regretfully a lifelong condition that is characterized by periods of remission and relapse. Treatment will need to be varied according to the position and severity of the lesions at any one time.

SELF-HELP GROUP

National Psoriasis Foundation
6600 S.W. 92nd Ave., Suite 300
Portland, OR 97223
503-244-7404
http://www.psoriasis.org
email: getinfo@npfusa.org

Pyloric Stenosis

ALTERNATIVE NAME

Congenital hypertrophic pyloric stenosis. (This alternative is a misnomer, because the word "congenital" implies a condition present at birth, whereas the symptoms of pyloric stenosis only very rarely begin before a child is 2 or 3 weeks old. Also, the condition has never been reported in a stillborn baby.)

INCIDENCE

The incidence of pyloric stenosis is four times higher in boys than in girls. It is thought that about 1 in every 250 male babies are affected, with a figure of 1 in 1,000 for girls.

Pyloric stenosis is most commonly found in Caucasian races and is rare in persons of Asian descent. Among Chinese babies, for example, the condition is virtually unknown.

Surgery for pyloric stenosis is one of the most common abdominal operations to be performed in the early weeks of life.

CAUSATION

While no direct genetic link has been found, there appear to be definite family factors at work. It is probable that a number of genes are involved and also that there is some sex linkage—the latter would explain the higher incidence in boys.

HISTORY

Until surgery became possible to relieve—and cure—pyloric stenosis, many babies succumbed to death. The obstruction to the passage of food into the intestine meant that starvation, dehydration, and severe electrolytic upset were the result.

The results of Ramstedt's operation for pyloric stenosis were first published in 1912, and soon after that time, the operation became routine procedure.

CHARACTERISTICS

The pylorus is that part of the stomach leading into the duodenum (the first part of the small intestine). It consists of a thick band of muscular tissue, which opens periodically to allow the contents of the stomach (where the initial processes of digestion take place) to pass into the small intestine, where further digestion and absorption takes place.

Hypertrophy (enlargement) of this muscular band effectively narrows the lumen of this canal; as a result, the emptying of the stomach is initially delayed and eventually ceases altogether. These facts lead to the symptoms.

Projectile vomiting starts when the baby is around 2 or 3 weeks old. The vomiting is violent and can be projected several feet. Immediately after vomiting, the baby will be anxious to feed again. This reaction is in direct contradistinction to vomiting due to an infectious process, where the baby will refuse to eat. As the condition progresses, **weight loss** occurs and the baby generally **fails to thrive.**

Constipation due to lack of any nutrients passing through into the intestine becomes evident within a few days. The baby with pyloric stenosis typically has a hungry, worried expression, which is hardly surprising when the basic necessities of life are missing!

Diagnosis can be confirmed by observing a **swelling** that passes across the top of the baby's abdomen as a feeding is given. The swelling can be seen and felt.

X-ray studies used to be done to confirm the diagnosis, but today **ultrasound** is the preferred diagnostic method.

MANAGEMENT

Ramstedt's operation, performed under general anesthesia, is safe and has excellent results. In this procedure, the enlarged muscle of the pylorus is divided, allowing fluids to pass uninterrupted through to the small intestine. Babies will be able to feed normally within three to four hours following the operation, and they are usually allowed to go home after 24 to 36 hours. After the surgery, feeding is best done with the baby in a sitting position, and leaning toward the right. This position will assist in the emptying of the stomach.

Before Ramstedt's operation became an option, antispasmodic drugs were used, with generally unsatisfactory results. They have no place in modern treatment.

COMPLICATIONS

If the vomiting has been severe and prolonged before surgery, **irritation of the stomach lining** can occur. This condition can, at times, cause post-operative vomiting.

THE FUTURE

There are no known after-effects in later life due to pyloric stenosis in infancy, although some authorities have suggested that the incidence of peptic ulcer is higher than normal for persons who suffered from the condition as babies.

Rashes

INCIDENCE

No overall incidence can be quoted, as there are a multitude of different causes for a rash. Every single child has probably had some kind of rash at some time during childhood.

CAUSATION

The causes of skin rashes can be divided into two broad categories. Some rashes are associated with, and part of the signs of, other illnesses. The infectious fevers of childhood are good examples of this type. Then there are all the rashes that arise in the skin itself with only little, if any, involvement of the rest of the body.

Rashes differ in their appearance according to the cause. There are five different types of rash:

- **macules,** which are flat lesions that have a pink or red color and cannot be individually felt;
- **papules,** which are round, raised, and red and so can be easily felt when running a hand over the surface of the skin;
- **vesicles,** which are round, raised, and filled with fluid, which can be either clear, or opaque because of pus formation;
- **petechiae,** which are spots rather like small bruises and do not whiten when pressed with a finger—larger areas of this type of rash are termed **purpura;**
- other, more **specific rashes,** as seen in eczema or fungal conditions.

Each condition having a rash as part of the disease will have one or other of these types of rash; for example, macules and papules often appear together.

CHARACTERISTICS

Rashes associated with a wider illness

The following infections all have a **maculopapular** rash (a mixture of macules and papules) as part of the features of the condition: measles, rubella, scarlet fever, fifth disease, roseola infantum, and Kawasaki disease.

The position of the rash on the body and the rash's timing are distinctive for each of these illnesses; other symptoms will be specific to the individual condition. Rashes can be a part of some viral infections that have no specific symptoms other than general debility, loss of appetite, and possibly a cough and a runny nose. The rash disappears as the infection clears.

Conditions that have a rash consisting of **vesicles** are chicken pox and some allergic conditions.

Petechiae is associated with the serious condition meningococcal meningitis. Henoch–Schönlein purpura also has this type of rash—as the name implies.

All these conditions are described individually in other parts of this text.

Rashes associated only with the skin

There may be a mild constitutional upset with these conditions, but usually it is only the skin that is affected.

Impetigo (discussed in its own entry) and **molluscum contagiosum** both have macules or papules as the specific rash. Molluscum contagiosum is a rash most commonly seen among 2- to 5-year-old children, and is due to a pox-type viral infection. The rash is discrete, round, and pearly white in color. It most usually arises in the armpit area and down the sides of the chest. This infection is transmitted from child to child when swimming or by siblings sharing a warm bath. The child is not at all unwell, and the rash will eventually clear spontaneously. Showering instead of bathing and temporarily avoiding swimming will prevent re-infection and the prolongation of the rash.

Eczema, pityriasis, and **psoriasis** have very specific types of rash, all of which tend to have a very scaly surface. (These conditions are described elsewhere in the text.)

Ringworm and *Candida* **infection** are two relatively common skin rashes that are both caused by a fungus. Ringworm is—as the name suggests—a circle of small bright-red papules surrounding a white center. This infection can be picked up from pets such as dogs, cats, and hamsters, as well as cattle—and other children. There is no added constitutional upset with ringworm, but treatment with antifungal creams is necessary to prevent its spread—both across the individual's body and also among other children (and adults). *Candida* (yeast) is a common fungal infection often found in young babies in the mouth or the diaper area.

(Further information on *Candida* can be found in the entry on diaper rash.)

There is one further unusual skin infection, which is caused by a specific bacteria of the staphylococcal strain. This infection is known as **staphylococcal scalded skin syndrome (SSS)** because of the rash's striking resemblance to skin that has been scalded by hot liquid. The appearance of the skin in this condition is quite unlike any other condition with a skin rash. Fortunately, only the superficial layer of the skin is involved, so fluid loss—a dangerous side effect of a severe scald—is not a problem. The child will, however, be in a good deal of pain with this infection and will also run a fever. Within a week, the top layer of skin will peel off, leaving normal skin without visible scarring. Penicillin is needed to treat this condition, and powerful painkillers are usually needed in the initial, acutely painful stage.

Rashes in children are notoriously difficult to diagnose, but the associated symptoms can make the picture clear within a few hours or days. Inquiries into similar symptoms in other members of the family will often be a help with rashes due to infectious disease.

Roseola Infantum

ALTERNATIVE NAMES

Sixth disease; three-day fever; exanthum subitum.

INCIDENCE

The exact incidence of roseola infantum is not known. It probably occurs more frequently than is reported, as the symptoms can be easily confused with a number of other conditions that are also associated with a rash. It is a disease of infancy.

CAUSATION

Roseola infantum is caused by a virus—the human Herpes virus 6. It is possible to confirm the diagnosis by cultivation of the virus from the blood of affected children. This test is rarely done, however, as the disease runs a brief course with only very few instances of complications. Diagnosis is made clinically by the characteristic symptoms.

CHARACTERISTICS

The infection begins suddenly with a relatively **high fever**—between 102° and 105° Fahrenheit. The child will have **little appetite** and will feel generally **unwell** and **irritable,** especially when the fever is at its height.

The fever lasts for three to five days and then the temperature falls suddenly back to normal. As the fever drops, a **rash** appears. It is a discrete red rash that occurs mainly on the **torso and neck,** although the arms, legs, and face can also be involved. In direct contrast to measles, there are **no signs inside the child's mouth** of a specific rash, although there may be ulcers on the tongue and soft palate. Also, again unlike measles, the rash does not coalesce but remains as **discrete markings** on the skin.

In addition to these signs, the **lymph glands** at the back of the neck are often enlarged. This sign can make the differential diagnosis from rubella difficult—and indeed, the two conditions are frequently confused. The age of the child and the sudden onset of high fever before the rash appears, however, should make clear the diagnosis of roseola infantum.

INVESTIGATIONS

An uncomplicated attack of roseola infantum usually requires no further investigation, the diagnosis being made from the signs and symptoms. If blood is taken, tests will show a rise in the white blood cell count during the days when a fever is present. A viral study can be done, but that is not a routine procedure.

MANAGEMENT

There is no specific treatment for roseola infantum. The main risk is that a **febrile seizure** can occur, due to the sudden rise in temperature. If a seizure does occur, attempts need to be made to **cool the child:** remove all excess clothing; avoid hot, stuffy rooms; and sponge the child down with tepid water. Seizures should also be reported to the child's doctor, who may prescribe a **sedative** to be given if the seizure recurs.

Apart from treatment for that complication, a **light diet** with **plenty of fluids** and an appropriate drug to help lower the temperature—such as **acetaminophen**—are all that is needed.

COMPLICATIONS

Complications are rare, the main one being a febrile seizure, as described above. In very rare instances, **encephalitis** (when the infection affects the brain) can occur. Here, the child will not make the usual quick recovery; instead, she or he will become progressively more ill and will have seizures. Medical aid under these circumstances is urgently needed.

PREVENTION

There is no vaccine available for roseola infantum. Immunization would seem unnecessary for such a comparatively benign disease with few serious complications or side effects.

THE FUTURE

There are no long-term sequelae due to roseola infantum, apart from the extremely rare effects of encephalitis.

Rubella

ALTERNATIVE NAME

German measles.

INCIDENCE

The true incidence of rubella is exceedingly difficult to determine because many cases of this infection are so mild as to pass unnoticed. From studies on antibody levels to the infection in adult populations, it is thought that around 90% of urban dwellers were infected with rubella in their youth—many of these people probably never realized that they were affected. People who live in more rural areas have a lower incidence because of their decreased likelihood of meeting the infection.

It is probable that rubella is primarily a disease of childhood, the infection most probably being acquired between the ages of 5 and 12 years.

HISTORY

Rubella has been known for many years. The rather unfortunate name of "German measles" came about because of the early descriptions of the infection in Germany, and because rubella has a slight, superficial resemblance to measles. In fact, rubella is no more common in Germany than anywhere else, and it certainly has no relationship at all to measles! It was only in 1962 that the rubella virus was finally identified and cultured—a surprisingly late date for so common a disease.

This mild disease can have devastating effects on fetal development if a woman contracts the infection during the first three months of pregnancy. These effects were discovered through brilliant detective work by an Australian doctor in the 1960s.

CAUSATION

Rubella is caused by a virus. The incubation period of the infection is between 14 and 21 days.

CHARACTERISTICS

The typical **rash** is often the first sign of the disease in children. The rash begins on the face and rapidly spreads over the chest, back, and, to a lesser extent, the limbs. The rash is fine and pink, with the spots in some cases becoming so extensive that they coalesce. The length of time that the rash persists varies considerably. The rash is usually apparent for up to five days, but it can last merely a few hours or not appear at all.

Swelling of the **lymph glands** in the neck is a constant feature of infection with the rubella virus. This enlargement can precede the appearance of the rash. The swollen glands can be tender. In fact, the first clue that a rubella infection is present is often tenderness on the neck felt when a child's hair is brushed.

Mild fever, headache, and general **malaise** can accompany the infection, but in many cases, the child may not feel any ill effects of the disease.

MANAGEMENT

There is no specific treatment for an attack of rubella, and, indeed, treatment is rarely required because of the mild nature of the disease.

Analgesics may be necessary for headache and fever control—in appropriate dosage and type for the individual child. (Aspirin compounds should not be used for children under the age of 12 years, because of the possibility of Reye syndrome.)

Children should be **kept away from school** during the acute stage of the disease when the rash is in evidence or they are feeling unwell. With a fleeting rash and a mild infection, it can be difficult to know that a child is infected, but if there is any suggestion that a child may have rubella, the **school should be informed** so any teachers who are pregnant can then take steps to determine whether or not they are immune to rubella.

COMPLICATIONS

Rubella has a very low complication rate. A transient **arthritis** can occur in the small joints of the body—hands, wrists, and ankles, in particular. This condition occurs more frequently in adults suffering from the disease, but can also occur in children.

Encephalitis (inflammation of the brain) can occur following rubella, but this complication is very rare.

Epistaxis (nose bleeding), **hematuria** (blood in the urine), or **purpura** (small bleeding spots under the skin) can also occur in association with an attack of rubella, due to changes in the blood from the infection. These conditions will resolve without specific treatment.

PREVENTION

Rubella is a disease that is preventable by **immunization.** From a public health standpoint, it is important that the highest levels of immunization are reached in order to reduce to a minimum the number of babies born with "rubella syndrome," a devastating condition in which babies are born deaf, blind, and/or with a heart condition because their mothers contracted rubella during the first three months of pregnancy. By ensuring that the pool of infection among young children is reduced, there is less likelihood that rubella will infect pregnant women.

Immunization against rubella is given as part of the **MMR** (measles, mumps, and rubella) injection to children between the ages of 1 and 2 years old and again later in childhood, usually before a child enters school. Rubella immunization is also available to those women who lack immunity to rubella.

THE FUTURE

There are virtually no long-term effects following an attack of rubella, apart from the possible effects on the newborn baby if a woman contracts rubella during her pregnancy. It is to be hoped that a time will arrive when no more babies are born with rubella syndrome, as a result of the elimination of this particular infection.

Scabies

INCIDENCE

Scabies is an infestation with a mite. It occurs worldwide and is especially common in the developing world and in places where hygiene is less than perfect.

Scabies is unusual in that there appears to be wide fluctuations in incidence. Epidemics seem to arise about every 15 years or so. In recent years, the incidence of scabies has markedly increased, perhaps because a form of natural immunity to the mite that develops among communities is on the decline.

HISTORY

Scabies has been known since the 17th century. It is said to be the first human disease for which the cause was known—i.e., infestation with the mite *sarcoptes scabiei.*

CAUSATION

Infestation with a specific mite is the cause of the symptoms. The adult female scabies mite is only around half a millimeter long, and its appearance has been described as closely resembling a minute tortoise. The female mite stands on her head to gain entry into the human skin and then burrows parallel to the surface of the skin. As the mite travels along, she lays eggs. These burrowing activities leave S-shaped tracks, which are visible to the naked eye and are typical of the condition. It can be difficult to see the tracks as they are so small and are also frequently obscured by skin inflammation due to scratching.

CHARACTERISTICS

Scabies is characterized by intense **itching,** which is worst at night when the body is warm. The irritation not only affects the places where the mite is active, but can occur all over the body. The pervasiveness of the irritation is thought to be due to the body's generalized hypersensitivity to the presence of the mite.

The appearance of the **rash** associated with scabies can vary considerably. For example, raised blistered spots can be seen alongside raised red discrete spots, all overlaid with scratch marks caused by the afflicted person's attempt to quell the overwhelming irritation. As a result of scratching, the skin can become infected. With all these various lesions on the skin, it can often be very difficult to find the "burrows" of the scabies mite that is the basic cause of all the problems.

The **most usual sites** for scabies to occur are around the insides of the wrists, under the arms, between the fingers, and around those areas of the body where clothes fit tightly—such as the waist and the groin. Other areas of the body can also show signs of the infestation, but usually the palms of the hands, the soles of the feet, the face, and scalp regions remain clear. (One exception to this latter statement occurs when the infestation affects young babies. In these infants, the face and hands are often also affected.)

The diagnosis of scabies is often delayed because of the difficulty of finding the typical burrows of the scabies mite among all the possible differing lesions on the skin. The marked irritation should arouse suspicion, especially if more than one member of the family—or a nursery school class—is having this problem. The infestation is passed on from person to person by close physical contact. Scabies cannot be "caught" from clothing or bedding.

MANAGEMENT

There are a number of preparations available with which to treat scabies. Permethrin is probably the best known and most effective medication. This emulsion should be applied to the whole of the child's body, with the exception of the head and neck. It should be applied following a warm bath and allowed to dry on the body. Treatment should be given on two consecutive nights to ensure that all the mites—in all stages of development—are eradicated. If there is a good deal of secondary infection as a result of frequent and persistent scratching—which can be almost impossible to control—an appropriate **antibiotic** will need to be prescribed. The **whole family** may need to be treated if there is any suggestion that they too are affected. Nightwear and bed linen will need to be laundered in the usual way following treatment with permethrin in order to remove its unpleasant odor from the fabric.

Unfortunately, the itch may still persist for several weeks after treatment. A specific cream is available that will help to control this unpleasant aspect of the condition.

Schooling can continue as usual once the treatment has been undertaken.

Scarlet Fever

INCIDENCE

The exact incidence of scarlet fever is not known, but the infection is certainly far less in evidence than it was 50 years ago. At that time, scarlet fever was a much-dreaded disease, both because of the severity of the illness itself and because of its possible complications—rheumatic fever and glomerulonephritis. These complications were frequently seen because of the absence of any specific treatment for scarlet fever.

Over time, the virulence of the bacteria causing this infection appears to have diminished, making the disease less serious when it does occur today than it was in the past.

Scarlet fever is an uncommon condition among preschool children.

HISTORY

Between the two world wars, fever or isolation hospitals were an integral part of the health scene. Patients, both children and adults, were nursed in these isolation units in an attempt to control the spread of infections. Scarlet fever patients formed a large segment of the populations of these fever hospitals. Today, antibiotic treatment has replaced the need for such isolation facilities.

CAUSATION

Scarlet fever is caused by a particular strain of the group A beta-hemolytic *Streptococcus* bacterium. (Beta-hemolytic *Streptococci* are classified according to the changes seen when the bacteria are grown under laboratory conditions.) These bacteria are also among the organisms that cause the skin infection impetigo.

The bacteria are usually passed from child to child by droplet infection. They can also be passed via contact with a wound, burn, or skin infection contaminated with the particular bacteria. The incubation period is a short one: one to seven days is quoted, but symptoms usually appear three to five days after contact with the bacteria.

CHARACTERISTICS

Scarlet fever usually starts very abruptly with the sudden onset of:

- **a headache;**
- **a very sore throat;**
- **a fever,** which can be very high for the first few days of the illness;
- **vomiting.**

These features can also be seen at the onset of any severe throat infection or tonsillitis. It is when the typical **rash** of scarlet fever appears, usually on the second day of the illness, that a definite diagnosis can be made. The rash is typically one of a generalized redness (or erythema) of the skin, with specific small spots of an intense scarlet color (hence the name of this condition). The rash begins on the face and rapidly spreads to the neck and chest and then to the limbs. Armpits, elbow creases, and the groin all show a dense concentration of the rash. Also, the rash on the face is quite typical, as the area around the mouth is free of the bright red rash.

The rash starts to fade after two or three days. In severe cases, the skin where the rash has been at its height begins to peel off, leaving clear skin underneath. Mild attacks do not show this desquamation process. (In the past, this peeled skin was much feared, as it was thought to carry the infection. It is now recognized that the shed skin is sterile.) With the disappearance of the rash, the young patient will begin to feel better. The fever will drop; the sore throat and headache will disappear; and appetite will improve. The **tonsils** and whole throat will be reddened, with white patches covering the surface. **Ears** can also be affected and are seen to be reddened.

The appearance of the **tongue** is quite unique in scarlet fever. It is initially coated with a white, fur-like substance, through which the bright red spots of the infection show. At this stage, the condition is termed "white strawberry" tongue; in a couple of days, the whole tongue becomes red—"red strawberry" tongue.

INVESTIGATIONS

If diagnosis is uncertain, throat swabs can be taken and sent to the laboratory to determine the infectious organism. This procedure is rarely done, as scarlet fever can so readily be diagnosed from the clinical signs and symptoms.

MANAGEMENT

Antibiotic treatment has transformed scarlet fever from a serious disease, with the possibility of long-term complications, to a relatively mild, although unpleasant, illness. Penicillin is the antibiotic usually prescribed to treat this infection, but erythromycin can also be used for children who are allergic to penicillin.

Within 48 hours of starting treatment, there is no longer any possibility of passing on the infection to another person.

It is important that the antibiotic treatment is continued for ten days in order to completely eradicate the bacteria. There is no need to give penicillin as a prophylactic measure to other children in the family, unless they are taking steroids for some other condition. Under those circumstances, they should be given penicillin to ensure that they do not suffer an attack from the *Streptococcus* bacillus.

Analgesics—usually in the form of some acetaminophen compound for children—can be given to relieve headache and sore throat. This drug will also help to lower the temperature, making the young patient feel more comfortable.

A **light diet** with **plenty of cool fluids** is helpful during the stage of the acute sore throat. The child will usually have little, or no, appetite for solid food, but it is important that adequate fluids should be given to prevent dehydration, which can occur, especially if the fever is high.

Bed rest for the first two or three days, when the temperature is at its height, will probably make the child as comfortable as possible. As soon as the child wishes to get up, quiet play in a warm room is quite satisfactory.

Schooling can be resumed as soon as the child's general health and energy have returned to normal (i.e., when the rash has completely disappeared, the throat is no longer sore, and a normal appetite and interest in usual activities have returned).

COMPLICATIONS

With immediate and adequate treatment with penicillin, or other appropriate drug, complications are uncommon.

Acute otitis media, in which there is earache and redness on examination of the eardrum, can occur as part of the initial symptomatology. Penicillin will rapidly cure this possible complication.

Sinusitis and/or **enlarged neck glands** can occur following scarlet fever.

In the pre-antibiotic era, **glomerulonephritis** often occurred a few weeks or months following the primary illness. In this condition, the kidneys can be seriously damaged and leave the affected individual with long-term problems. This complication rarely, if ever, happens today. Similarly, **rheumatic fever,** which frequently affected the heart, was once a feared complication of scarlet fever, but it is virtually unknown today. **Bronchopneumonia** is another once-common complication, but antibiotics ensure that this condition rarely develops nowadays.

PREVENTION

There is no immunization available against scarlet fever. The causative organisms, *Streptococcus* bacteria, are to be found in 10 to 20% of the throats of perfectly healthy children. With such a widespread finding, immunization would be difficult, and as the treatment is so relatively easy and successful, there would not seem to be the need for a vaccine. Early diagnosis and treatment are the mainstays to prevent the serious complications of the disease.

THE FUTURE

An attack of scarlet fever, as discussed above, rarely leads to any long-term complications these days. One attack does not necessarily lead to immunity from acquiring a sore throat with *Streptococcus* as the causative organism, but individuals rarely develop full-blown cases of scarlet fever more than once.

Sleep Disturbance

INCIDENCE

Problems with nighttime waking and difficulties in getting a child to sleep at bedtime are extremely common. Recent research has indicated that up to 20% of 2-year-olds wake in the night at least five times every week. Boys and girls seem to be equally affected.

Subjectively, it would seem that only a very few fortunate parents have no problem at all with the sleeping patterns of their children.

CAUSATION

Illness of any kind, even the common head cold, can give rise to sleeping difficulties—this observation is true for anyone of whatever age. A stuffy nose and an irritating cough are not conducive to quiet sleep, and a fever will make anyone restless.

The **temperament of the child** has a bearing on sleep patterns. The overactive child will have as much difficulty falling asleep as she or he has controlling overactive behavior during the day. At the other end of the scale, quiet children may find that the "worries" of the day prevent sleep.

Parental anxiety regarding sleep can adversely affect the child's ability to settle down satisfactorily at night. Parents who frequently check on the child throughout the evening will only aggravate the feelings of insecurity regarding sleep that may be affecting the child.

Stressful events during the day can also play on a child's mind and prevent sleep. This problem can arise if, for example, a much loved grandparent has recently died. The child can be afraid that if he or she goes to sleep under these circumstances, he or she may also die.

CHARACTERISTICS

Sleep problems fall into two main groups: **difficulty in getting to sleep** and **frequent waking** during the night.

Both types of problems can give rise to much parental concern. Parents may feel that they have no time at all to themselves if their child will not go to sleep at a reasonable time. Frequent waking, too, can lead to complete parental exhaustion if the problem continues for months on

186

end. The child can make up for lost sleep during the day, but exhausted parents do not usually have this option.

Other sleep problems include the following.

Nightmares: These are unpleasant dreams that cause the child to awaken screaming in fright. The dream will be vividly remembered, and much reassurance is needed to calm the child and induce sleep again.

Night terrors are quite different from nightmares. In the case of a night terror, the child will awaken terrified, but she or he does not respond when spoken to and, at times, even seems not to see her or his parents. This altered state of consciousness can last for up to ten minutes, with the child being quite unable to be comforted. Eventually, sleep will return, and the child will wake in the morning with no recollection of the night's events or the distress that was so obviously felt at the time of the terror. Night terrors most frequently affect children between the ages of 4 and 7 years.

Sleepwalking is another sleep disturbance that usually affects older children—from around the age of 8 years into the teen years. The child gets up from bed with a fixed, blank expression, does not respond to anyone, and walks downstairs or into another room for no apparent reason. It is difficult to waken the child under these conditions, and rousing him or her should not be attempted (see below). The sleepwalker will eventually return to bed, and he or she will be quite unaware the following morning of the events of the night.

MANAGEMENT

Difficulty in getting to sleep can be helped by a **calm bedtime routine**—not necessarily an easy task for parents, who may also have meals to prepare and older children needing attention. A warm bath, a final drink, and a (non-exciting) bedtime story are ideal. This routine should be followed by a calm but firm tucking in and "good night." Requests for "a drink" or "to come downstairs" need to be firmly resisted. Once such disruptions are allowed, the pattern can be hard to break. Following a bedtime routine can be especially difficult following an illness where the child has obvious reasons for being unable to sleep. Any illness, of course, will need specific and appropriate treatment.

Nighttime waking can be due to any number of causes, and efforts will need to be made to sort out the individual reasons why the child wakes up. Perhaps she or he is disturbed by a specific noise at some time of the night? Or perhaps the lack of general household noise during the evening is a factor? It is surprising how comforting sounds of activity in other parts of the house can be when dropping off to sleep. A **nightlight** can reassure a child who wakes for some reason during the night. Again, any possible illness will need to be found and treated.

Children who have nightmares need reassurance that the unpleasant experience was only a dream and not a reality. A cuddle and the continuing **presence of an adult** until the child sleeps again are all that is needed. Recurrent nightmares should alert parents to the fact that there is some factor in the child's daily life that is causing concern. Some activity or particular events at daycare or school may need to be explained to the child or altered. Each individual child will react in a different way to the day-to-day events of everyday life.

Night terrors can be more difficult to handle. Again, identifying **potential stressful activities** during the day can help. Parents also find it reassuring to know that the child has no recollection of the nighttime fears. Children with night terrors will eventually outgrow these experiences.

Sleepwalkers need to be **protected from injuring themselves** during their perambulations—for example, parents should gently guide the sleepwalker away from stairs or pieces of heavy furniture that could cause injury. The sleepwalker should be led back to bed without any attempt being made to wake him or her. Sleepwalking occurs during the phase of deepest sleep, and waking in a strange, unexpected place can be frightening. Any anxieties during the day need to be unearthed and discussed with the child.

THE FUTURE

Sleep problems do not affect all children. When problems do arise, however, they give parents cause for much concern—and weariness! Most sleep difficulties will be overcome by late childhood. There is no evidence to show that children with sleep problems have similar difficulties in later life.

Sternomastoid Tumor

ALTERNATIVE NAMES

Torticollis; wry neck. (These names are not true alternatives, as there are a number of other causes of torticollis. For example, a developmental abnormality in one of the vertebrae in the neck or a severe lymph node infection will give rise to a similar picture. Both these alternative names are, however, frequently applied to the condition.)

INCIDENCE

The incidence of this relatively mild condition has not been reported, but it seems to appear with a fair degree of regularity. It is more common in babies who have had a breech birth. Boys and girls are equally affected.

CAUSATION

Causation is unknown, but the relationship between a breech birth and a sternomastoid tumor is well documented. In fact, the tumor was once thought to be due to the trauma of a breech delivery. More recent studies suggest, however, that the abnormality exists prenatally and is possibly the cause—and not the outcome—of breech birth.

CHARACTERISTICS

The basic abnormality is found in one of the sternomastoid muscles in the neck. These muscles link the bony mastoid process behind the ear to the top of the sternum, and they function to turn the head. With a sternomastoid tumor, part of the muscular tissue of this structure is replaced by fibrous tissue, which effectively reduces the ability to turn the head. This abnormality is not dangerous to health, nor is it likely to spread to any other part of the body. Parents usually notice this condition when their baby is around 2 or 3 weeks old. The baby is seen to be **continually looking upward,** with her or his **head tilted** to one side. When the neck is examined, a **hard swelling** is found in one of the sternomastoid muscles.

MANAGEMENT

Physical therapy needs to be started as soon as possible after diagnosis. Exercises consist of gently rotating the baby's head to stretch the affected muscle.

Surgery may be required if the condition is missed in early life or if treatment fails to achieve a satisfactory result. Without adequate treatment, the child's face and neck will develop asymmetrically and the underlying structures in the neck may possibly become involved.

THE FUTURE

With adequate and successful treatment there are no deleterious after-effects from a sternomastoid tumor.

Sudden Infant Death Syndrome (SIDS)

ALTERNATIVE NAME

Crib death.

INCIDENCE

The incidence of this tragic event varies widely among countries and over time. In the USA during the 1980s, the incidence was 1.5 for every 1,000 babies born. This incidence made SIDS the most common cause of death for infants between 2 weeks and 1 year old. In Hong Kong, the incidence was much lower (0.2 for every 1,000 live births), while in New Zealand the incidence was higher (3 to 4 babies for every 1,000 born). No satisfactory explanation of these differences has been given.

Since the late 1980s, much attention and research has been directed toward possible causes and ways of prevention of SIDS. Increased awareness of the condition has resulted in a dramatic decrease in the number of babies found unexpectedly dead in their cribs.

A number of other features are important when looking at the incidence of SIDS. The most common age for this tragedy to occur is between 2 and 3 months old. Very few deaths due to this cause occur in the first two weeks of life, and after a child reaches the age of 7 months, the danger is lessened: only around 10% of SIDS deaths occur after this age.

Boys are more likely than girls to die in this way.

There is also a seasonal incidence, with more deaths happening in the winter months. (This finding may have something to do with the higher incidence of upper respiratory tract infections at this time of the year. A small proportion of babies were found to have had symptoms of a mild viral infection in the days immediately before death.)

SIDS occurs in all socioeconomic groups, but there appears to be an increased risk with deprivation; risk is also apparently greater for babies of women who have borne many children, children of young mothers, and babies with low birth weights.

Given all these facts, it is likely that there are a number of causative factors involved in the unexpected SIDS death of a young baby.

HISTORY

Sudden infant death syndrome has been described from time immemorial. It was once usual to attribute such deaths down to either "overlaying" or a deliberate act on the part of one or other parent. ("Overlaying" was the term applied to the supposed suffocation of the baby by parents—often thought to be drunk—rolling over on to the baby sleeping in the same bed.) It was only during the latter half of the 20th century, when more babies slept by themselves in cribs, that it became clear that sudden unexpected death did occur for reasons other than over-laying. However, the actual causes of death were unknown in spite of detailed postmortem examinations.

CAUSATION

As mentioned previously, there is no one known factor that can be definitely associated with SIDS. There are, however, a number of baby-care practices that have resulted in the fall of the incidence of this devastating condition.

Sleeping position of the baby: It is advised that babies are laid to sleep on their backs or on their sides and not face downward—the supine (or face upward) position being preferable to the side position. This simple practice appears to be the most important action in reducing the number of babies suffering a crib death.

Tobacco smoke: Parents—and visitors—are advised not to smoke anywhere near a young baby. Also, mothers are advised not to smoke at all during pregnancy. Exposure to tobacco smoke is considered to be the single most important avoidable factor related to SIDS. (Children raised in nonsmoking households also have fewer upper respiratory tract infections than those children whose parents smoke.)

Overheating has been suggested as a possible cause for SIDS. In today's centrally heated homes, babies do not need warm pajamas or multiple bed coverings. It must be remembered that babies cannot move and throw off excess coverings if they feel too hot.

Breastfed babies appear to be less at risk of SIDS than babies fed on formula. It is possible that some form of allergy may be a factor here.

Mild infection is also thought to be a possible factor, although most babies with infections survive them with no problems. Parents, however, are advised to contact their doctor if they are at all worried about their young baby's health—particularly if the child is younger than 7 months old.

Regrettably, **nonaccidental injury** must always be remembered as a possible cause of SIDS.

MANAGEMENT

In this context, "management" refers to the sequence of actions that need to be taken after the unexpected death of a baby. After their devastating discovery, parents typically contact either their own pediatrician or the emergency department of the local hospital. The baby will be examined, and parents will be asked to remember, if possible, the sequence of events that led up to the time when they found their baby dead. This case history should include any worries the parents may have had regarding the baby's health the day or two before of his or her death.

It is important that parents are given the chance to hold their dead baby, as this opportunity does much to aid the normal grieving process. In all instances of SIDS, a **postmortem examination** must be carried out. This procedure can seem unnecessary—and upsetting—for parents, but it is important that any known cause of death is identified. Relatives and / or friends should be contacted before the parents return home, and a medical social worker can be of comfort and support at this time.

Later contact can be arranged, if the parents wish, with local **SIDS parental support groups.**

It is also important that parents are given a chance to **discuss events** two or three weeks later with their baby's pediatrician. Many anxieties and questions will have arisen over this time that need discussion and clarification.

At a later date, if another **pregnancy** is considered, parents will need much support. Fears of a recurrence are always present when caring for another young baby.

PREVENTION

At present, factors that have reduced the incidence of SIDS are:

- putting babies to **sleep face upward;**
- **avoidance of tobacco smoke**—both before and after birth;
- **avoidance of overheating;**
- **breastfeeding;**
- careful checks on minor episodes of **illness** when babies are at the critical ages.

THE FUTURE

Research is continuing in many parts of the world on all aspects of sudden infant death syndrome.

SELF-HELP GROUP

Sudden Infant Death Syndrome Alliance
1314 Bedford Avenue, Suite 210
Baltimore, MD 21208
410-653-8226 or 800-221-7437
http:/www.sidsalliance.org
email: sidshq@charm.net

Temper Tantrums

INCIDENCE

Every child has probably had at least one temper tantrum in the early years of life. Tantrums can be isolated incidents, or they can occur more frequently as part of wider behavioral problems.

Both sexes seem to be equally affected, and the usual age group affected is between 18 months and 3 to 4 years old.

CAUSATION

Between the ages of 18 months and 3 years, children's verbal and physical skills are developing fast, as are their desires to handle objects, behave in more "grown-up" ways, and attempt tasks beyond their physical competence. When these facets of development do not agree, a temper tantrum can result. **Frustration** or **simple injuries,** occurring when a child attempts a too difficult task, can be precipitating factors.

Other factors can be involved in the frequency and severity of temper tantrums. **Physical disability** or **chronic illness** can give rise to greater degrees of frustration. The child sees peers behaving in a way that highlights his or her disability—a potent reason for venting anger.

Parental difficulties, such as marital disharmony or parental illness, can have profound effects on a child's perceptions and reactions. As he or she attempts to gain security, a temper tantrum may be the only way possible for a child to express feelings. Poverty or other forms of **social deprivation,** including the consequences of poor parenting skills, can have a similar effect.

A child's specific **temperament** will also have a bearing on the range of the temper tantrums. The quiet, easy-going child will feel no need to express him- or herself in this way. Other children with more outgoing, and perhaps more aggressive, personalities will be more prone to these outbursts.

CHARACTERISTICS

These can vary widely, but everyone has seen, and felt sympathy for, the young parent struggling with a load of groceries and a screaming and kicking toddler lying on the floor of the supermarket. More aggressive children will fly at siblings or parents, physically attacking their targets but only very rarely hurting themselves in the process!

Holding one's breath is a specific—and frightening—form of temper tantrum. Again, these incidents are usually precipitated by anger, frustration, or an emotional upset. The child cries for a few minutes and then holds his or her breath and stops breathing. The child's face will turn blue, and, on occasions, he or she will lose consciousness and fall to the ground. Jerking movements of the limbs can follow, and it is a difficult to determine whether or not the child is experiencing an epileptic seizure or a simple breath-holding attack. With a breath-holding attack, however, recovery is quick and complete, whereas the child who has had a seizure will be drowsy and confused for a time.

Somewhat similar, but even more alarming, are **reflex anoxic seizures,** in which the child becomes suddenly extremely pale and limp, and loses consciousness. Recovery is rapid—within one minute—and complete. Again, this event can follow from some minor injury, such as a bumped head or a scratched knee. These attacks are due to the over-activity of a specific nerve in control of the pulse. There is often a familial tendency to these worrying attacks.

MANAGEMENT

Most temper tantrums are self-limiting, the child ceasing the antisocial activity and starting to cry quietly. It is important that parents should recognize their child's need for reassurance and affection at this time. That can be a difficult task, considering the troubles through which the child has just put her or his parents! However, it must be remembered that the child, too, is overwhelmed by previous feelings of anger or frustration and can feel very frightened by the strength of the emotions he or she experienced.

It can be necessary to **restrain a child** in the throes of a temper tantrum because of the possible physical danger he or she may pose to self or to other people. The best way to restrain a child is to fold arms around the child's body from behind and so stop flailing arms and legs from creating mayhem. Avoid giving excess attention to the child in a tantrum; instead, praise should be given when behavior is good.

Breath-holding attacks and **reflex anoxic seizures** need to be **discussed with a doctor,** particularly if twitching of the limbs has occurred during these attacks. It is important to distinguish between these attacks and an epileptic seizure. A good description of the events before the attack can be helpful in clarifying the diagnosis.

Reflex anoxic seizures may continue throughout early childhood and can be frequent. Treatment with **atropine** has been found to be effective if these occurrences are too frequent, but this drug must be prescribed by the child's doctor.

THE FUTURE

Temper tantrums are usually outgrown by the time school days start, coinciding with children's increased ability to express themselves and their feelings.

Tics

INCIDENCE

It is thought that the rapid, repetitive, involuntary muscular movements known as tics affect up to 10% of the childhood population. Children between the ages of 7 and 12 years are most commonly affected. Boys outnumber girls three to one in these habits. There is frequently a family history of tics. Some tics do persist into adult life.

CAUSATION

Frequently, a child who has a tic faces a **stressful home or school situation.** It would seem that the tic develops almost as a superstitious ritual against stress in these circumstances. **Imitation** is also a powerful stimulus to the development of a tic. A classmate with twitchy eyes, or a grandparent with a limp, can often be found in the child's immediate environment.

Simple tics must be differentiated from chorea and Tourette syndrome. In **chorea** (a symptom seen in a number of illnesses, including a type of cerebral palsy, or following encephalitis, for example), the movements are not so stereotyped and predictable as with tics. **Tourette syndrome** is a particularly distressing ailment where there are many violent, complex muscular tics, which are sometimes associated with the repetition of obscene words and an odd form of barking cough. This syndrome is extremely difficult to treat and, unlike common tics, continues into adult life in around 50% of cases.

CHARACTERISTICS

Tics can affect any part of the body, but they usually involve the head and neck areas. **Blinking** of the eyes, **twisting of the mouth,** and/or **shrugging of the shoulders** are among the most commonly noted tics.

In a tic, the group of muscles that are involved in each series of movements is always the same, so that one is aware in advance of exactly what will happen next. (This finding is in direct contradistinction to involuntary movements due to other physical causes.)

Repetitive coughing, swallowing, or sneezing are other forms of tic found in children. These tics often begin under circumstances of acute embarrassment for the child, then continuing when the particular stress is removed.

MANAGEMENT

Most cases of tics resolve spontaneously given time, but it is thought that about 6% of children with tics will still have their specific tic as adults.

Parents should be advised **not to grumble at or ridicule** their child with a tic. Such reactions are counterproductive, only drawing attention to the problem.

Family therapy can help where there are family tensions and anxieties. Pediatricians will be able to give advice on how to contact skilled people to undertake this therapy. **Behavioral therapy** is also helpful. Therapists can show parents techniques to distract the child's attention when the tic is manifest.

Tranquilizers can be tried a last resort, particularly if the child is overactive in addition to having a tic. These drugs must be carefully controlled, however, and never continued for any length of time.

THE FUTURE

The majority of simple tics resolve themselves by the time children become teenagers. A few adults will still have their tics throughout their lives, and these will become part of their individual personalities.

Tics caused by chorea or Tourette syndrome have a less successful outcome than other types and need specialized treatment.

Tonsillitis

INCIDENCE

There are no figures of exact incidence available for this unpleasant infection of the throat, but every pediatrician will see several children every week with tonsillitis, particularly during the winter months. Preschool and early school-age children usually suffer from three or four upper respiratory infections during the course of any one year. While all these infections are by no means tonsillitis, a significant number of them will involve the tonsils. (The pharynx, housing the tonsils at either side, is closely allied to the middle ear. Infection frequently occurs in both these parts of the body simultaneously—but for descriptive purposes, it is best that ear and throat infections are discussed separately.)

Boys and girls are affected equally, and tonsillitis is seen in all races.

CAUSATION

The tonsils are two masses of lymphoid tissue situated at the back of the throat, and in children under the age of 8 years old, they are relatively large even when they are clear of infection. Tonsils fulfill the function of dealing with bacteria and viruses before these invaders have the chance to proceed to the lower respiratory tract (i.e., the lungs and associated structures). As the tonsils perform their work dealing with infection, they become red and swollen. During this process, pain is felt and there is also a generalized constitutional illness.

Tonsillitis can be caused by either bacteria or viruses.

CHARACTERISTICS

Fever is one of the first and most common signs of tonsillitis. The fever can be high, particularly in young children, and it sometimes gives rise to a febrile convulsion. (A febrile convulsion is a seizure caused by the reaction of the immature brain to a high body temperature. Such seizures rarely occur in children over the age of 5 years.)

Children over the age of 5 years are more likely to complain of a **sore throat** than those who are younger than 5. The younger children frequently complain of a **stomach ache** rather than a sore throat. In both age groups, there will be a **reluctance to eat**.

When one looks down the throat of the sufferer, the cause of the problem will become obvious. The tonsils are **red and swollen.** In really severe infections, the two tonsils appear almost to meet in the midline of the throat, which explains why the child is refusing food!

Swollen glands in the neck are also a frequent feature of tonsillitis. These cervical glands drain infection from the back of the throat, and in so doing, they become enlarged and tender. A **blocked, stuffy nose** can also accompany an infection in the tonsils. The congestion is due to associated infection in the adenoids—masses of lymphoid tissue situated at the back of the nose, which also become swollen and inflamed by the infectious process.

The child with tonsillitis will feel generally **unwell** and miserable.

INVESTIGATIONS

Tonsillitis is diagnosed by the clinical signs and symptoms. A throat swab sent to a laboratory can determine the causative infectious organism. In practice, however, this test is rarely done, as treatment needs to be started before the laboratory results become available.

MANAGEMENT

The acute attack

Penicillin is the antibiotic of first choice for an attack of tonsillitis; it will relieve unpleasant symptoms within 24 to 48 hours. It is important that the full course that has been prescribed should be taken, in order to eradicate fully the invading organism. If necessary, **acetaminophen** (in doses and strengths appropriate to the age of the child) should be given to relieve sore throat and headache. This drug will also help to lower the temperature.

For the first 24 to 48 hours of the infection, the young sufferer will only be willing to consume **fluids.** It is vital that sufficient fluid is given at this time. Children can quickly become dehydrated as a result of the high fever so frequently seen during an acute attack of tonsillitis.

Bed rest is not essential, unless the child feels more comfortable tucked in bed. Quiet play in a warm room with the chance to lie down when tired is usually a favored option for a young child with an acute attack of tonsillitis.

Tonsillectomy

This operation has had its fashionable periods: tonsils were very readily removed for slight reasons in bygone days. Today's criteria for this operation are more rigid. Most ear, nose, and throat surgeons would only consider removing a child's tonsils if:

- the child has suffered from more than three attacks of confirmed tonsillitis in one year over a two-year period; and/or
- the tonsils are so large as to meet in the midline even when an acute infection is not present. This state of affairs can be dangerous to normal breathing, especially during sleep.

Tonsillectomy is performed by an ear, nose, and throat surgeon under a general anesthetic. At that time, the surgeon will also consider whether or not removal of the adenoids is necessary. A stay of one or two nights in the hospital is the general rule. Children recover very quickly from the removal of their tonsils—far more rapidly than do adults undergoing this procedure. Cool fluids and a soft, easy-to-swallow diet for a day or two is all that is needed by way of post-operative care. For school-age children, a couple of weeks off school is advisable to ensure that additional throat infections are not contracted too soon after the operation.

THE FUTURE

If a child's tonsils have been chronically infected for a number of years, with frequent attacks of acute infection, she or he will benefit enormously from tonsillectomy. Appetite, energy, and general health will all improve, and growth will often show a spurt. On the down side, however, a tonsillectomy does not guarantee that sore throats are a thing of the past! Throat infections can—and do—still occur, but they are less frequent and recovery is quicker than they were before the surgery.

Toxocara

INCIDENCE

The incidence of infections with toxocara—a type of roundworm—is not precisely known. Infections with this parasite may be more common than is recognized, as a child's immunity can be built up before the condition is diagnosed.

CAUSATION

The *toxocara canis* worm is a normal inhabitant of the intestine of the young dog and the fox. These animals gain natural immunity to the parasite by around 6 months of age, when the adult worms are expelled from the hosts' bodies. Because of this immunity, no ill effects from the worms are seen in older dogs, although the worms may still exist in an encapsulated form. However, during pregnancy, bitches lose this immunity. Reinfection, or reactivation of the dormant larvae occurs, thereby affecting the unborn puppies, who are then born infected with the toxocara worm.

Children acquire the infection by swallowing the minute eggs of toxocara—either directly from the saliva of puppies, or from crawling around on carpets, lawns, and other areas where eggs may be deposited. As would be expected, younger children—especially those who are in the crawling years—are the most frequently affected age group. (At this age, too, children typically explore everyday objects putting them in the mouth.) When inside the child's body, the larvae (born from the ingested eggs) are unable to mature in the child's intestine—where, in the dog and fox, the worms normally find their home. Therefore, the larvae wander aimlessly around the child's body, setting up areas of inflammation in a variety of sites—the liver, kidneys, lungs, muscles, the brain, and eyes can all be possibly affected. (This wandering is known by the splendidly descriptive name of *visceral larvae migrans*.) It is also thought that the type of toxocara affecting cats—*toxocara catis*—causes similar symptoms.

CHARACTERISTICS

Signs and symptoms of infection with toxocara can be very diverse. In some cases, infection with toxocara may never be diagnosed because the child has a wide variety of nonspecific symptoms and may recover spontaneously. However, certain clues can help in diagnosis.

The child affected is typically between 1 and 7 years old, the time when children crawl and put many different objects into the mouth. At this age, also, hygiene is rudimentary!

There is frequently the arrival in the home of a new puppy prior to the onset of symptoms.

Signs and symptoms of infection can include:

- **failure to thrive adequately,** i.e., poor weight gain and lack of general growth;
- **pica:** a desire to eat all kinds of strange substances (earth, coal);
- a **low-grade fever;**
- a **cough,** with episodes of wheezing;
- **anemia;**
- **seizures;**
- **blurred vision,** with possible subsequent loss of vision due to involvement of the retina. The blurring is caused by inflammation of this vital part of the eye, and the possible subsequent loss of vision is caused by the detachment of the retina. Children with these ocular manifestations tend to be in the older age group— between 7 and 9 years old.

All these symptoms will not occur in any one infected child. The symptoms will depend on which organ, or system of the body, is involved in the infection.

Untreated, the infection runs a slow, benign course with the child's natural defense mechanisms eventually overcoming the infection. Usually within 18 months, full health is restored.

INVESTIGATIONS

Blood tests will show if any anemia is present, and blood samples can also be used for serological testing to determine if antibodies against toxocara are present. (It is interesting to note that up to 7% of adults show positive results to this latter test. This finding implies that they were infected by toxocara at some time or other in their earlier life. Obvious symptoms may not have occurred, but the adults with positive test results have successfully overcome the infection.)

MANAGEMENT

In many cases, the diagnosis of toxocara is uncertain for some time, and the child's very general and nonspecific symptoms are treated empirically. For example, antibiotics are given for the cough and iron medication for the anemia. These medicines will result in improvement in the child's general health, as there can be added infection in the respiratory tract or an iron-deficient anemia as a result of a poor appetite.

Once investigations have proved that infection with toxocara is present, there are several specific drugs that can be used with success, although treatment may take several weeks. Steroids can also be used to advantage to reduce the inflammation at various sites in the body.

COMPLICATIONS

The most serious complication is the loss of vision that can result from the migrating larvae in the eye. There are specific drugs available to treat this condition and to help preserve vision.

PREVENTION

Infection of children with toxocara has evoked much "anti-dog" publicity in recent years, but two points must be remembered.

First, infections of all kinds abound in our immediate environs, and toxocara is just one of them. With care and good hygiene, this infection can be contained at least as readily as many others.

Second, pets of all kinds are valuable to both children and elderly people. Children learn responsibility and facts about biology as they attend to their pets' needs. Lonely and upset children in particular can gain much comfort from a pet.

A few sensible precautions will, however, need to be taken to ensure that the risk of toxocara infection of young children is reduced to a minimum.

Dogs should be wormed regularly with the appropriate medication, which is available from vets.

Children should be taught not to allow dogs to lick their faces and to wash their hands thoroughly after touching their pets and before eating.

Dog owners should control their dogs at all times and should not allow them to foul public walkways or open spaces.

Communities should ensure that it is not possible for dogs to foul parks, sand boxes, or other places where children are encouraged to play.

If these precautions are observed, toxocara infections could be eliminated without the need to destroy or ban all pet dogs.

Tuberculosis

INCIDENCE

In developed countries of the world, incidence of tuberculosis (TB) has declined rapidly since the middle of the 20th century, although there has been a recent resurgence of TB with the increasing prevalence of HIV infection. The decline is due to better living conditions and less overcrowding, as well as better treatment of known cases of tuberculosis. "Contact tracing," and subsequent treatment, if necessary, of people who live or work in close proximity to a sufferer, has also done much to reduce the incidence of tuberculosis. Nevertheless, this infectious disease remains an important problem, especially as a drug-resistant form of TB that is especially hard to treat spreads among certain populations.

People living in unhygienic conditions are at increased risk of contracting this disease.

Worldwide, it is estimated that there are between 3 and 4 million new cases of infectious tuberculosis every year, and there is probably an equal number of people who have smear-negative (or noninfectious) tuberculosis. The figure for children suffering from tuberculosis worldwide is around 1.25 million cases every year. Half a million children will die from the disease annually.

Recognizing the difference between infectious and noninfectious cases of tuberculosis is important for understanding how the disease spreads. In infectious cases, the sick person coughs up the infecting organism, which can thus be passed to other children and adults. These cases are known as "smear-positive," as the offending bacteria can be isolated from the infected person's sputum. Noninfectious people can have the disease in any number of systems of their bodies, including the lungs, but they do not cough up the organism. They are therefore known as "smear-negative," as their sputum does not contain the tuberculosis bacillus.

When infection with tuberculosis has occurred, the body becomes sensitive to the protein contained in the bacillus. This sensitivity shows itself in a positive skin reaction when a special preparation of the purified protein derivative (PPD) of the tuberculosis bacterium is injected into the superficial layers of the skin. This procedure is the basis for the Mantoux and Tine tests described below.

CAUSATION

Tuberculosis is caused by a bacteria of the *mycobacterium* genus, and it was first described by Dr. Robert Koch. The infection can be transmitted in milk from infected cows, as well as from person-to-person. Transmission through milk no longer occurs in developed countries because all herds of dairy cows are tuberculin-tested to ensure that they are free from this disease.

CHARACTERISTICS

The initial infection with tuberculosis occurs in the lungs. This primary focus can subsequently progress in two different ways.

On settling in the lungs, the bacteria will multiply here (usually in the upper part of one or the other lung). The lymph nodes draining the affected part of the lung will also become involved in the infection. This group of involved tissues is then known as the **primary complex.** This infection can easily pass unnoticed; occasionally, the child will run a low-grade fever and be vaguely ill for a week or two. The body's natural defenses are mobilized and seal off the infected area of lung. It is at this stage—which is reached within four to six weeks—that the skin tests for tuberculosis become positive. The lesion in the lung is usually too small to be visualized on an X-ray, although the inflamed lymph nodes around the area can often be seen.

The primary infection that proceeds along these lines is not infectious to anyone else. Later in life, this primary focus can become reactivated. The tuberculosis bacillus can remain dormant for many years. Symptoms can occur when the bacteria is released from its dormant position when the body's resistance is lowered by another illness, a general decline in health, or some other cause.

The second type of progression occurs if the child is poorly nourished, ill with another intercurrent infection, taking immunosuppressant drugs for some other condition, or in generally bad health. Under these circumstances, the initial infection with the tuberculosis bacteria can spread through the blood to a wide range of other tissues in the body, including further invasion of the lungs.

In the lungs, extensive destruction of lung tissue can result, making the child seriously ill. There will be a **fever,** a **persistent cough,** and **night sweats.** Fortunately, this picture is rarely encountered in the USA today, but it must be remembered when investigating this classic triad of symptoms.

The TB bacillus can invade the **meninges** (the delicate tissue covering the brain and spinal cord), giving rise to **tuberculous meningitis.**

Symptoms of this infection will be those seen in all types of meningitis—headache, vomiting, and fever. Lumbar puncture, obtaining a sample of cerebrospinal fluid for laboratory analysis, will determine which organism causes the symptoms.

Bones can also be affected by the spread of the bacteria. The spine is the most usual site affected, closely followed by knees and/or hips. The affected site will be painful, and X-ray changes will confirm the diagnosis.

Lymph nodes, especially those in the neck, can also become infected with the TB bacillus. Initially, these infected glands will be enlarged but not tender (as they are with a throat or ear infection). Later, if untreated, these swollen glands may break down and emit discharge.

Other organs, including the **intestines, kidneys,** and **larynx,** can be affected, although these sites are rarely infected in children in Western countries today.

All these latter aspects of spread from the primary focus are uncommon in developed countries. However, in other parts of the world, where poverty and disease are rife, these problems are not rare.

INVESTIGATIONS

X-ray of the chest, or other parts of the body where suspicious symptoms occur, will usually show the typical lesions of tuberculosis.

A **Mantoux** or **Tine test** (described below) will also be positive if the infection is due to the tuberculosis bacterium. The extent of the reaction to these tests will point to the range of activity of the infection.

MANAGEMENT

The "primary complex" is often not treated, as it frequently passes unnoticed. Even if the child is slightly feverish and ill for a short while, the true cause of the malaise is rarely discovered. Some authorities suggest that known primary-focus cases should be treated in order to prevent spread of the disease. (It must be emphasized that the primary focus is not infectious.)

Treatment for other forms of tuberculosis belongs to a highly specialized area of medicine. There are a number of **drugs** available to treat tuberculosis infection today. These drugs will need to be continued for some length of time—up to 12 to 18 months—in order to eradicate the disease. The child, of course, must be carefully monitored throughout this time, both for success of treatment and for possible adverse side effects from the drugs used.

Attention to **living conditions** must also be of paramount importance in the successful management of tuberculosis. Adequate and appropriate **nutrition** of the sick child (and, in many cases, the immediate family as well) can require attention. **Contact tracing** of other members of the family and close social contacts must be carefully undertaken.

Schooling can be continued if the child feels well enough to cope with the demands of school. Arrangements for home tuition may well be necessary during the early stages of treatment, depending on the site and severity of the infection.

COMPLICATIONS

These have already been discussed in the section on the generalized spread of tuberculosis.

PREVENTION

Prevention is by **immunization** with the Bacille Calmette–Guérin (BCG) vaccine, which was first produced in 1921 by the Frenchmen Calmette and Guérin. There is little clinical indication for the use of this vaccine in the USA, but it is widely used in developing countries where the prevalence of TB is much higher. Use of this vaccine can make the PPD and Tine tests positive decades later, even though the person was never actually infected with TB.

The BCG vaccination, if it is indicated, is given intradermally into the upper arm. The vaccine will result in a small spot within two to four weeks. The spot can sometimes ulcerate and discharge, taking up to three months to heal. Children who have a malignancy or an immunological disease and children who are on steroids should not receive the BCG vaccine.

Tuberculosis is an infection against which vigilance must be maintained. In many parts of the world, it is still a potent killer, especially of people with HIV. Rapid and adequate tracing of contacts of all cases of known tuberculosis is the first line of defense.

THE FUTURE

Old tuberculosis infection in the lung can be **reactivated** in later life if, for some reason, the body's defenses are reduced. It is vital that both the sufferers and their immediate contacts should receive quick and appropriate treatment.

Urinary Tract Infection

INCIDENCE

Urinary tract infections are more common in childhood than was thought a few decades ago. The signs and symptoms are often so nonspecific and intermittent that the problem is not diagnosed.

The prevalence is estimated to be between 1 and 2% in girls, but below 1% in boys. (In infancy, as many boys are affected as girls.) A general practitioner will probably see at least two or three children every year who have a new urinary tract infection. That may not seem an enormous number, but it is important that the diagnosis is made and the condition treated adequately to prevent further problems for the individual child in later life.

Urinary tract infections can be the first clue that there are **abnormalities in the renal tract.** These abnormalities if undiscovered—and hence untreated—can give rise to problems later in life.

CAUSATION

Urinary tract infections are caused by bacteria. The type of bacteria involved are usually those found normally in the gastrointestinal tract where they do no harm. The *E. coli* bacteria is one of the most common types involved. Infection of the renal tract is usually prevented by the natural defense mechanisms of the body. For example, any bacteria gaining access to the bladder are regularly washed out by the flow of urine. Also, the child's natural immune defenses preclude the infection gaining a hold in the renal tract. Breakdown of the natural defense mechanism can be caused by urine remaining in the bladder for relatively long periods of time, which, in turn, can be due to a number of factors:

In around 40% of the cases of children with recurrent urinary tract infections, X-rays show a **vesicoureteral reflux,** in which urine is refluxed back into the ureters. The phenomenon is thought to have its origins in a congenital defect in the anatomy at the junction of the ureters into the bladder.

Any **obstruction** to the normal outflow of urine from the bladder can cause an infection. **Folds,** or **valves,** in the urethra can cause this type of obstruction, as can **stones** in older children.

Incomplete emptying of the bladder can also have a bearing on the amount of urine that remains in the bladder for long periods of time. Children often say they have "finished" using the toilet, when, in fact, a great quantity of urine remains in the bladder. (At school, the bladder may be emptied infrequently—perhaps due to a dislike, or fear, of school toilets. This practice can cause the bladder to over-distend and subsequently to empty incompletely.)

The causative factors in the onset of urinary tract infections are complex and are intricately interwoven. Various tests, interpreted by skilled personnel, are necessary to unravel these factors in each individual child.

Girls are more at risk of infection than are boys due to the relative shortness of the female urethra.

CHARACTERISTICS

Urinary tract infections are notoriously difficult to diagnose in children because signs and symptoms can be vague and nonspecific, and often seem unrelated to the urinary tract. The younger the child, the more non-specific will be the symptoms.

Classically, the symptoms associated with a urinary tract infection are:

- **burning pain when passing urine;**
- **pain** either in the **lower abdomen** or higher up in the **loin** region if the infection has reached the kidneys—when it is known as a **pyelonephritis;**
- **frequency** in the passage of urine;
- **enuresis** and/or daytime wetting;
- the passage of **blood in the urine** (hematuria).

This picture is more usually seen in the older child with a urinary infection.

Younger children are more likely to be suffering from a urinary infection when:

- there is a **failure to gain weight** adequately;
- the child is generally **irritable,**
- her or his bad mood is associated with a **poor appetite;**
- there is a **low-grade fever,** or spikes of fever perhaps with an associated febrile convulsion;
- **vomiting** occurs with no previous obvious stomach upset.

Examination of a sample of urine will either confirm, or exclude, a urinary tract infection.

INVESTIGATIONS

In order to carry out a **urine test,** it is necessary that a clean sample (i.e., one that is not contaminated with either bacteria from the surrounding skin or by feces) is obtained. To obtain a clean sample, the middle of the stream of urine should be taken. An uncontaminated sample is easier to obtain from boys than from girls, but with care, and after cleansing of the perineum, a clean sample can be obtained from a small girl as she sits on the toilet. Younger children can be fitted with a special bag until sufficient urine is obtained—again, of course, after thorough cleansing of the perineum.

The urine should be examined under the microscope as soon as possible after collection—within an hour if left unrefrigerated. (Refrigeration for 24 hours is satisfactory for later laboratory examination.) Pus cells, white blood cells, and bacteria can be visualized under the microscope if they are present.

Another method of value in the general practice situation is to use a special **dipstick,** which is a plastic strip coated with special chemicals that change different colors in the presence of different substances in the urine, such as blood or protein.

Blood tests will show a raised white blood cell count and ESR if an infection is present.

If a urine test proves infection to be the cause of the child's symptoms, further investigations (after the treatment of the acute attack) should be carried out in order to see if the **kidneys** have been involved in this, or previous, infections, and to detect any **abnormalities in the renal tract.**

There are a number of specialized tests available. Different authorities usually prefer one test over another. The type of investigation pursued in the case of any one child will also depend on the facilities available locally. The following investigations are possible.

X-ray examination of the abdomen, as a preliminary examination, will determine whether any defects in the spine are causative factors in the onset of the urinary tract infections. Any calcium stones in the urinary tract will also be revealed in an X-ray.

Ultrasound investigation can discern any obstructive problems and can be used to measure bladder capacity and function.

A doctor may also perform a **voiding cystourethrogram,** in which a radiopaque dye is passed up into the bladder; as the dye is subsequently voided from the bladder, X-ray pictures are taken of the process. This procedure is a particularly useful investigation in the detection of vesicoureteral reflux. Also, any congenital kidney abnormalities—such as "horseshoe" or "duplex" kidneys—will be detected, and the extent of any scarring of the kidneys from previous infections can be seen.

Isotope scanning (DMSA scan) is another investigation that is available at some centers. This specialized investigation is especially valuable in determining the presence and/or extent of kidney damage.

Intravenous pyelogram can also be used to give a comprehensive image of the structure and function of the whole urinary tract. This procedure involves an intravenous injection of a radiopaque substance.

Not all these investigations will, of course, be necessary in any one individual. Local availability, medical preference, and the duration and severity of symptoms will all be taken into account when investigations are planned.

Sexual abuse must always be remembered as a possible source of recurrent urinary tract infections, and a watch must be kept for other signs and symptoms of this sad situation.

MANAGEMENT

The acute attack

Babies and children with severe urinary tract infections will need hospital treatment. Older children and those with milder attacks can be treated at home.

Antibiotics will need to be given as soon as possible. The choice of antibiotic will depend on the type of organism causing the infection. It is not necessary, or wise, to await laboratory results before starting treatment. A wide spectrum antibiotic can be used until sensitivities are available. The type of antibiotic can always be changed if it is found that a different one is more appropriate for the specific infection. Children who are seriously ill, or who are vomiting frequently, will need to be given antibiotics intravenously. Seven days of antibiotics should clear the infection.

Plenty of **fluids**—and an **analgesic** if pain is a problem—will help to lower temperature and reduce malaise.

Future management will depend on the results of the investigations undertaken. For example, if any obstruction to the flow of urine, such as stones, is found, it will need to be treated.

PREVENTION

Further infections must be prevented as far as possible to avoid long-term effects. **Bubble bath** should be avoided in the baths of children susceptible to urinary tract infections. The surface-tension lowering action of these products aids the entry of bacteria into the bladder.

Other preventative measures include:

- giving a long-term dose of antibiotics. The length of time that these drugs should be given is variable, but a minimum of two years is advised by most authorities;
- ensuring that the child empties her or his bladder fully. Drinking plenty of water and allowing adequate time for visits to the toilet are two important measures. Avoiding constipation is also helpful—overloading of the large bowel can exert pressure on the lower urinary tract and effectively prevent adequate bladder emptying;
- assessing progress at follow-up appointments, with further investigative procedures when necessary. These procedures are vital to be sure that a low-grade infection does not persist, as well as to encourage child and parents to persist with treatment. (Long-term medication can be trying for everyone concerned.)

COMPLICATIONS

Recurrent urinary tract infections, with the continuing risk of further renal damage, are an ever-present worry.

Renal failure can occur if damage has been severe in childhood. **High blood pressure** can also be a late result of earlier kidney problems. **Kidney function** is intimately related to hypertension, but early, adequate treatment of urinary tract infections in childhood can eliminate at least one possible cause of this problem.

Urinary tract infections in childhood are an excellent example of how adult disease often has its basis in the early growing years.

Warts

ALTERNATIVE NAME

Verrucas.

INCIDENCE

Warts are common skin lesions, especially during childhood. In fact, almost all children will have warts somewhere on their bodies before they reach adulthood.

Plantar warts, which are found on children's feet, reach almost epidemic proportions at times. This type of wart is rarely seen in persons after the age of 16 years.

HISTORY

Warts have been mentioned in history from time immemorial. Probably one of the best-known characters in British history with facial warts is Oliver Cromwell, who had a splendid crop. It is only in recent years that a greater interest has been shown in these benign tumors of the skin. The causative factor—a particular type of virus—is known and is seen to multiply rapidly in the nuclei of cells. It is recognized that under certain circumstances, infection with one of the viruses causing warts can lead to malignant change. Further study of warts may help to unravel aspects of malignancies in the body.

CAUSATION

Warts are caused by one of the Papilloma viruses—of which there are many—of the Papova group. It is thought that the incubation period (the period between infection and the appearance of the wart) is long.

CHARACTERISTICS

Four different types of wart are described; it is possible that a different type of subgroup of virus is involved in each type.

The **common wart** or **verruca vulgaris** is most usually seen over bony surfaces such as knees and elbows. Small, regular episodes of minor injury to these parts of the body may allow the virus to gain a hold. These warts are raised, and under a magnifying glass they can be seen to have an irregular, bumpy surface.

Plane warts are, as their name implies, flat and are usually found on exposed parts of the body, particularly the face. They are also seen to occur along the margins of scratches and cuts—frequently in large numbers.

Plantar warts—usually referred to merely as "verrucas"—are found on the soles of the feet. In recent years, much publicity has been given to this type of wart because of the high number of children acquiring them from swimming pools, and also following barefoot exercise and dancing. Plantar warts can become large and exceedingly painful from the trauma of continually walking on them.

Warts around the anus and genital regions of the body tend to have a frilly, fronded appearance. The possibility of sexual abuse must always be investigated when a child is found to have warts on this part of the body.

MANAGEMENT

Management can be fraught with difficulties. For example, numerous plane warts on the face can be very difficult to treat. Plantar warts, too, can be numerous and cover a large, much-used part of the foot. The fact that warts frequently occur in groups also makes treatment difficult. Furthermore, warts quickly appear out of the blue, and at times they disappear with equal rapidity. (Many are the old wives' tales connected with this phenomenon—one of the best-known being that if you rub the wart with raw steak and then bury the steak in the garden, as the meat degenerates, so too will the wart disappear!)

Specific treatments include the following.

Paints, which basically remove hard skin, can be applied to the wart on a regular daily basis. It is preferable that the painted area is covered by an adhesive bandage to avoid rubbing off the paint. This treatment will need to be continued for some time, and it frequently fails because affected persons quit using the paint too soon. Paints are available without a prescription.

Podophyllin can be used when a person has only a few warts, or only one. It should be applied daily and covered with a dressing. This substance must be used with caution, however, as it is extremely irritating when applied to normal skin. Between applications, the surface of the wart can be gently rubbed away. Podophyllin is available only with a prescription.

Liquid nitrogen can also be used for isolated warts. Again, it is important that the wart should be treated accurately, as surrounding normal skin can be easily damaged.

Soaking the feet daily in a solution of **formaldehyde** used to be a favorite treatment. Following each soak, the surface of the wart was gently pared away. This is slow, long-term treatment, and it is rarely used today.

Warts can be **cauterized.** A local anesthetic is injected around the wart, and the warty tissue is burnt away. Care must be taken not to damage the surrounding skin. It is unwise to use this method for warts arising over joints or on the palms of the hands or soles of the feet. The resultant scars can be painful in these specific locations.

A simple, but often effective, method for the solitary wart is merely to cover it with an **airtight bandage**. This procedure effectively cuts off the oxygen supply to the wart. After two or three weeks of this treatment—changing the bandage at bath times, or as and when it becomes dirty or loose—the wart will become soft and friable. It can then be gently scrubbed off with pumice or an ordinary nailbrush.

PREVENTION

Preventative methods are only possible with plantar warts—the ubiquitous verrucas that are passed so readily from child to child in the warm, moist atmosphere of swimming pools. A few authorities still inspect children's feet before swimming, excluding from the pool those children found to have a verruca. This screening process is difficult to implement fully, and perhaps not entirely reasonable to enforce. No child ever died from a verruca, but many children have lost their lives because they were unable to swim. **Verruca socks** have had their vogue in the past and are still available. Children don these foot coverings before entering the changing room (where most of the infections are passed on) at swimming pools.

Warts are a nuisance rather than a danger. However, there are occasions when treatment for these irritating lesions becomes necessary. Painful verrucas on feet, disfiguring marks on the face, or warts on fingers that get in the way of daily activities are all examples of reasons for active treatment. Even with conscientious treatment, warts can be particularly persistent. Their only saving grace is that they will eventually disappear spontaneously within a year or two if left alone!

Whooping Cough

ALTERNATIVE NAMES

Pertussis; the "cough of a hundred days."

INCIDENCE

The incidence of whooping cough showed a marked variation in the last decades of the 20th century. The variation is closely related to the administration of whooping cough vaccine: the incidence was dramatically higher when immunization rates were low, and it fell as immunization against this vicious disease became more acceptable.

Whooping cough is known worldwide, and in the mid–1980s there were approximately 60 million cases annually, with half a million deaths reported annually. Without immunization, it is thought that by the age of 5 years, 80% of children are infected. Epidemics of this infection occur once every three to four years. (It is thought that whooping cough is underreported in most countries where standardized reporting systems are in place. The true incidence of this disease is probably very high indeed.)

Whooping cough is unusual among the childhood infections in being more common, and more severe, in girls than in boys.

CAUSATION

Whooping cough is caused by a bacterium, which is spread by droplet infection from a child already suffering from the disease.

The mode of action of the whooping cough bacterium (*Bordetella pertussis*) is unusual. The bacterium itself first attacks the respiratory passages, producing the initial symptoms of the disease, which are rather similar to those of a common cold. The bacterium then produces a toxin that attacks various cells throughout the body. While the initial bacterial attack is susceptible to, and can be treated with, antibiotics, these drugs will have no effect on the later toxin.

The incubation period of whooping cough is 7 to 14 days—10 days being the average time before the next family member starts to show symptoms.

CHARACTERISTICS

Whooping cough is a long illness, with three distinct phases.

During the **catarrhal stage,** symptoms closely akin to a common cold occur—a **runny nose,** a **cough,** and a **mild fever.** This stage can be so comparatively mild that the child may still be at school or playing with her or his peers. As she or he is infectious at this time, the disease can be quickly spread.

The **paroxysmal stage** follows after about ten days. In this stage, the cough occurs in severe spasms, and the child has great difficulty in getting adequate breath between the paroxysms. The face will become puce and even blue as the child seeks to get air into the lungs, and the paroxysm will end in a "whoop" as the air is finally drawn in a rush into the lungs. Once heard, the whoop of whooping cough can never again be forgotten. **Vomiting** frequently occurs at the end of the paroxysm of coughing, particularly if the child has just eaten. These paroxysmal attacks are extremely distressing to both parent and child. With closely repeated paroxysms, the whole family—and especially the sufferer—can become completely exhausted. This phase can last up to two weeks. The lack of oxygen experienced by the child during these paroxysms of coughing can be the cause of one of the most serious of the complications of whooping cough. The severity of the paroxysms can result in **hemorrhages** into various parts of the body—into the conjunctiva of the eyes, from the nose, and even small bleeding areas into the skin.

During the **convalescent stage,** the cough gradually decreases in both frequency and severity, but it can still be in evidence up to three months later—hence the name, "the hundred-day cough."

If the disease occurs in a young baby, the characteristic whoop is often absent because the baby will not have the strength to take the large gasp that is the cause of the typical whoop.

INVESTIGATIONS

The diagnosis of whooping cough is essentially a clinical one, and a very obvious one once the whoop is heard. If there is a current epidemic of whooping cough and a child has a persistent, worsening cough lasting for longer than two weeks, whooping cough can be strongly suspected.

Blood tests will show a nonspecific increase in certain white blood cells.

Laboratory tests on the secretions obtained from the back of the nose and throat can confirm the diagnosis. Such tests, however, are rarely done, partly because of the unpleasantness for the child of the procedure involved in obtaining a sample of these secretions, and partly because of the unreliability of some of these tests.

MANAGEMENT

A specific antibiotic, **erythromycin,** is given to destroy the bacteria (but with no action against the toxin produced). This treatment will also render the child noninfectious after around five days. The erythromycin should be continued for two weeks to eradicate all the bacteria.

During the unpleasant paroxysmal phase, the child can be helped in a number of ways. Efforts should be made to **avoid provoking the paroxysms** of coughing. For example, sudden changes of temperature can initiate an attack, so staying in a warm, evenly controlled environment can be helpful. Similarly, bland food that does not irritate the back of the child's throat should be offered.

Meals should be small and frequent. If a fit of coughing results in vomiting, with the loss of most of the previous meal, food can be offered again once the attack is over. The child will often be willing to eat again immediately after an attack of coughing. It is important to do everything possible to maintain the child's nutrition during the illness. Fluids should also be available in abundance to ensure that dehydration does not complicate the illness.

The **sticky mucus,** which is produced as part of this disease, **must be removed** from the child's respiratory passages as much as possible. This procedure is especially important in babies and young children, who find it difficult, or impossible, to cough up this mucus. (This aspect is one of the reasons why whooping cough is such a dangerous illness in the young child.)

Children with whooping cough can become very distressed and frightened during the paroxysms of coughing (as can the adults watching their child fighting for breath) and will need much **reassurance.**

Most older children can be **kept at home** through an attack of whooping cough. Young babies, or those children in difficult or unsuitable home circumstances, will need to be **hospitalized** during the worst of the illness. Hospital admission for a short time may also be necessary to relieve parents who are nursing several children through this long-drawn-out illness.

The child can return to **school** as soon as she or he feels well enough—as long as at least five days treatment with erythromycin has been given. It is unlikely, however, that the child with even a mild attack of whooping cough will feel well enough to return to school for at least two or three weeks. Teachers should be fully informed about the course of the illness—mainly because the cough, which can last for up to three months, can give rise to concern. Teaching staff should be reassured that the child is not infectious during this convalescent stage as long as erythromycin has been given.

COMPLICATIONS

As well as being a highly unpleasant, and potentially fatal, illness, complications are common with an attack of whooping cough.

Lungs

Bronchopneumonia not infrequently occurs along with an attack of whooping cough. Resistance is lowered by the effects of the whooping cough bacteria and the toxin produced, so that secondary infection is common. If pneumonia occurs, the child's general condition will deteriorate and there will be a rise in temperature. Treatment will be with another antibiotic.

Children who suffer from **asthma** will have added problems if they contract whooping cough. Indeed, this infection may bring a hitherto undiagnosed asthma to light. Once recovery from the whooping cough has occurred, appropriate treatment for the asthma must be given.

Some authorities think that an attack of whooping cough in childhood contributes to long-term damage to the lungs—**bronchiectasis** being a common sequel. Appropriate antibiotic treatment during the acute attack will do much to reduce this possibility.

Ears

Secondary bacterial infection giving rise to **otitis media** frequently occurs during the acute stages of whooping cough. Earache and a rise in temperature are symptoms of this complication.

Hemorrhages

Because of the excessive strain put on blood vessels during the paroxysms of coughing, hemorrhages into various parts of the body can readily occur. **Conjunctival hemorrhages, petechiae** (bleeding from small blood vessels under the skin), and **nosebleeds** have already been mentioned. **Hemoptysis** (coughing up of blood) from the respiratory passages can also occur and add to parental anxieties. These hemorrhages will all resolve spontaneously, although nose bleeds can sometimes be difficult to control. Hemoptysis should always be reported to the doctor.

Hernias

Because of the severity of the paroxysmal attacks of coughing, the pressure inside the abdominal cavity is raised. If there is already a hernia present—in boys most usually in the groin area—or if there is an incipient weakness in the muscles in this part of the body, an attack of whooping cough can exacerbate the situation.

Nervous system

It is the complications in the nervous system due to the whooping cough bacteria that are the most serious. These complications can result in long-term handicap. It is thought that there are two ways in which these complications can occur:

- as a result of the temporary oxygen lack to the tissues, including nervous tissue, from the paroxysms of coughing—anyone who has seen the cyanosis (blueness) of a child's face during a paroxysm will readily understand that tissues are starved of oxygen during those few minutes;
- as a direct result of the effects of the toxin produced by the whooping cough bacteria on nervous tissue.

These neurological complications can manifest themselves as **seizures** or **loss of consciousness.** If severe, the outcome can be **permanent brain damage,** resulting in a range of possible effects, including **paralysis, intellectual handicap,** and **death.**

Regretfully, there is no treatment that can prevent such tragedies occurring, apart from, of course, prevention by immunization with whooping cough vaccine.

PREVENTION

Whooping cough can be prevented by **immunization** with the pertussis vaccine. This vaccine is offered as part of the routine babyhood immunization schedule. According to this schedule, pertussis vaccine should be given together with vaccines against diphtheria and tetanus as the **"triple" vaccine** at 2, 4, 6, and 15 months and 5 years of age. If the whooping cough part of this triple vaccine has been omitted for any reason, it can be given as three doses of single pertussis vaccine at monthly intervals.

Contraindications to receiving this vaccine are few. If the child has a feverish illness when any immunization procedures are due, they should be postponed until recovery has taken place. If there has been a severe generalized reaction to a previous dose of the whooping cough vaccine, this part of the triple vaccine should be omitted in future. A severe reaction means a high fever (over 103° Fahrenheit) within 48 hours of the injection; seizures, anaphylactic shock, or prolonged, inconsolable screaming by the baby within 72 hours of the injection being given. These are all pretty dramatic occurrences, which should not be confused with lesser reactions, such as a mild fever or irritability for a few hours. These latter mild reactions can occur following immunization with the pertussis vaccine, but when compared with the possible effects of a naturally acquired attack of whooping cough, the benefits of immunization can be seen.

A severe local reaction to a previous immunization at the site of the actual injection is a contraindication. A severe local reaction is defined by a large area of redness and swelling—covering the front and side of the baby's thigh or much of the circumference of the arm, depending on where the injection has been given.

Asthma or eczema are not contraindications to receiving the whooping cough vaccine.

If the baby has had any seizures earlier in life, or there is a strong history of epilepsy in the immediate family, individual advice regarding must be sought from a doctor specializing in immunization problems.

THE FUTURE

The late effects of an attack of whooping cough will depend on any complications that may have occurred. For most children, an attack of whooping cough will be a dim, distant, albeit unpleasant, memory. For some unfortunate children, this infection will color the whole of the rest of their lives.

Appendix A: The Progress of Selected Infectious Diseases

INTRODUCTION

It must be emphasized that no two people are the same and the same disease can affect different people in different ways; therefore, the following information should only be treated as a guide.

CHICKEN POX

Days	Stage	Comments
	Incubation	14–17 days' duration
1–5	Rash crops	Crops of "blistery" spots arise every 2–3 days
1–6	Fever	Usually peaks on third day—can be up to 102° Fahrenheit
6–9	Rash scabs	Spots crust over

NB. All stages of the rash can be seen at the same time.

MEASLES

Days	Stage	Comments
	Incubation	10–14 days' duration
1–7	Conjunctivitis	Sore reddened eyes associated with photophobia
1–7	Fever	Up to 104° Fahrenheit—usually peaks on fourth day
1–7	Coryza	Runny nose
1–11	Cough	Harsh dry cough
2–6	Koplik's spots	To be found on inside of cheeks opposite the back molars—similar to grains of salt
4–9	Rash—discrete	Face, upper torso, and arms—becoming a confluent dense rash all over the body after about 1–3 days

RUBELLA

Days	Stage	Comments
	Incubation	14–21 days' duration
1–8	Malaise	
1–12	Lymph nodes	Tender enlarged glands at back of neck
4–7	Conjunctivitis	Mild only, with no photophobia
4–7	Coryza	Runny nose
4–7	Rash	Fine, pink discrete spots
5–8	Fever	Mild only, but may be up to 100.5° Fahrenheit on fifth day

SCARLET FEVER

Days	Stage	Comments
	Incubation	2–4 days' duration
1–5	Sore throat	Severe sore throat
2–7	Fever	Can be up to 104° Fahrenheit on third day
2–7	Rash	Bright scarlet in color

Appendix B: Glossary

Abdominal cavity   That part of the torso below the diaphragm, containing many important organs.

Alveoli   Lung tissue involved in gaseous exchange.

Anal fissure   Crack in skin around anus.

Analgesics   Pain-relieving drugs.

Androgens   Male sex hormones.

Aneurysm   Ballooning of an artery.

Anorexia   Loss of appetite.

Antibiotics   Drugs active against bacterial infections.

Anus   Ring of muscular tissue at lower end of large bowel.

Bronchiolitis   An infection in the smallest bronchi in the lungs.

Capillaries   The smallest blood vessels in the body.

Cataract   Clouding of the lens of the eye.

Cellulitis   Widespread inflammation of connective tissue.

Cerebrospinal fluid   Fluid surrounding the brain and spinal cord.

Chorea   Involuntary, non-stereotyped muscular movements.

Chromosomes   Units in every cell on which genes are situated.

Chronic   Long-standing.

Comedones   Plugs of hard skin found in acne.

Congenital   Conditions existing from birth.

Conjunctiva   Delicate tissue covering the eye.

Conjunctivitis   Inflammation of the conjunctiva.

Connective tissue   Tissues surrounding all the organs of the body.

CT scan   Computer-aided tomography.

Desquamation   Peeling of the superficial layers of the skin.

Developmental checks   Standardized tests used to check childhood development.

Diaphragm Strong sheet of muscle dividing the abdominal cavity from the chest cavity.

Dietitian Person trained in nutrition.

Droplet infection Spread of infection from minute drops of secretions in a person's breath.

EEG Electroencephalogram.

Elimination diets Diets used to exclude possible cause of an allergy.

Emollient creams Greasy ointments or creams used in skin diseases.

Encephalitis Inflammation of the brain.

Epicanthic folds Folds of skin over inner corner of some children's eyes.

Epiglottis Flap of tissue at the back of the throat controlling respiration and swallowing.

Epiglottitis Infection of the epiglottis.

Epistaxis Nose bleeding.

Erythromycin A particular type of antibiotic.

ESR (Erythrocyte sedimentation rate)—laboratory test used as an indicator of an infectious process.

Estrogens Female sex hormones.

Etiology The cause of, or factors involved in, the onset of a disease.

Eustachian tube Tiny tube linking the middle ear with the back of the throat.

Febrile convulsions Seizures seen in children under the age of 5 years due to a sudden rise in temperature.

Glaucoma Condition in which pressure inside the eye is raised.

Glycosuria Sugar in the urine.

Hemangioma A nevus due to an underlying abnormality in the blood vessels.

Hematuria Blood in the urine.

Hemoglobin Substance in red blood cells carrying oxygen.

Hemophilia Condition associated with defective clotting of blood.

Hemoptysis   Coughing up of blood.

Hernia   Weakness in muscular wall—usually of abdomen.

Hirschsprung disease   Condition in which there are narrowed segments of bowel.

Hormones   Secretions from ductless glands that are poured directly into the blood stream.

Hypertrophy   Enlargement of a part of the body.

Hypoglycemia   Low blood sugar.

Hypothermia   Low body temperature.

Immunization   Procedures eliciting a response in the body that protects against specific infections met at a later date.

Immunosuppression   A procedure whereby the immune system is suppressed by drugs in the treatment of certain diseases.

Incubation period   That period of time between exposure to an infection and the onset of symptoms.

Inhaler   Specialized equipment used to introduce medication into the lungs.

Jaundice   Yellow coloration of the skin due to malfunction of the liver.

Ketones   Substances that can arise from the breakdown of body tissue.

Koplik spots   Spots seen on inside of cheeks in the early stages of measles.

Labyrinthitis   Inflammation of structures inside the ears due to infection, causing vertigo.

Lumbar puncture   Procedure whereby cerebrospinal fluid is withdrawn for diagnostic purposes.

Lymph nodes   Congregation of lymph tissue in many different parts of the body.

Malaise   General feeling of illness.

Mastoid process   Bony projection of skull behind and below the ears.

Menarche   Time of onset of menstruation in girls at puberty.

Meninges   Thin, delicate covering of brain and spinal cord.

Meningitis   Inflammation of meninges.

Myringotomy   Procedure whereby an opening is made in the eardrum to withdraw fluid from the middle ear.

Nevi   Specific types of skin blemish.

Nebulizer   Equipment for introducing medication into the lungs by way of a face mask.

Orchitis   Inflammation of the testes.

Ossicles   Tiny bones in the middle ear—three in number.

Osteoporosis   Reduction in density of bones.

Otoscope   Instrument used for examining ears.

Pancreatitis   Inflammation of the pancreas.

Parasite   An organism living off another unrelated organism.

Parotid glands   Salivary glands situated in front of, and below, the ears.

Parotitis   Inflammation of the parotid salivary glands.

Petechiae   Small bleeding points under the skin.

Photophobia   Dislike of light.

Pica   Eating of dirt, or other unsuitable substances, e.g. coal, chalk.

Platelets   Part of the blood concerned with clotting.

Psychiatrist   A doctor specializing in mental illness.

Refractive error   Errors in the bending of light on to the retina.

Renal tract   Organs of excretion, consisting of kidneys, ureters, bladder, and urethra.

Retina   The structure at the back of the eye intimately concerned with vision.

Rheumatoid factor   Factor found in the blood of sufferers from some kinds of rheumatism or arthritis.

Rickets   Disease of bone due to lack of calcium and/or vitamin D.

Scoliosis   Sideways twist to the spine.

Sebaceous glands   Glands found all over the body producing sebum, which gives the skin its oily nature.

Septicemia   Bacterial infection of the blood stream.

Signing   Language using hand movements for deaf people.

Soft palate   Back of the roof of the mouth.

Syndrome   A combination of signs and symptoms which, when put together, form a recognizable pattern.

Thrush   A yeast infection of the mouth.

Tonsils   Aggregations of lymphoid tissue on either side of the throat.

Toxin   Substance produced by certain bacteria.

Trachea   Windpipe.

Ureters   Tubes connecting kidneys to bladder.

Urethra   Passage from bladder to exterior.

Vasculitis   Inflammation of the small blood vessels.

APPENDIX C: IMMUNIZATION

Immunization against some of the common childhood infectious fevers is one of the success stories of the 20th century. Before the introduction of vaccines, children had to suffer a naturally acquired attack (usually caught from another child) so that their immune systems could develop antibodies against the infection. With immunization procedures, the need to contract the specific infections (with all the attendant risks of complications and even death) is by-passed. Laboratory methods are available to modify the viruses and bacteria causing disease. Once an immunization is given, an immune response is possible without the toxic components of the infection that give rise to the unpleasant, and potentially fatal, symptoms of the naturally acquired infection.

There are two main forms of immunization—active immunization and passive immunization. By far the most commonly used method is active immunization, where modified organisms are injected (or given by mouth in the case of the polio immunization). This treatment stimulates the baby's immune system to produce antibodies against the specific organism that has been injected. These antibodies are then available to fight any future invasions of the body by the specific organisms.

Passive immunization is used less frequently and consists of an injection already containing antibodies. This type of immunization is used for short-term protection, such as overseas travel, or for children whose immune systems are compromised by existing conditions or by drugs to treat some other serious disease.

Immunization is an enormous and complex subject, and only a brief outline can be given here. For further detailed information, textbooks on immunization should be studied or a pediatrician consulted.

There are routine procedures for the immunization of all babies:

- at birth, 1 month, and 6 months, a hepatitis B vaccine is given;
- at 2, 4, 6, and 15 months, a combined vaccine against diphtheria/tetanus/whooping cough (pertussis) is given by injection as well as the injection against *Hemophilus influenzae* type b;
- also at 2, 4, and 6 months, the oral polio vaccine is given;
- at 15–18 months, babies are given a combined measles/mumps/rubella vaccine by injection and a varicella vaccine;

- at 3–5 years—booster doses of diphtheria/tetanus/pertussis and oral polio vaccines; a booster measles/mumps/rubella injection is also given;
- at 13–15 years—a booster dose of diptheria/tetanus vaccine is given.

The diseases against which immunization is available are potentially fatal and can leave behind serious, long-term handicaps. Therefore, while there are a few risks to immunization procedures, the benefits are enormous. Risks are reduced to an absolute minimum if the following contraindications to receiving the vaccine are observed:

- if the baby has an acute illness (immunization needs to be postponed until the infection has cleared);
- if a child has had a severe reaction to a previous immunization;
- if the baby has a condition in which the immune system is deficient; similarly, if the baby/child needs special medication to suppress his or her immune system for some other cause;
- if the baby has been born with a severe condition affecting his or her central nervous system.

Parents need to discuss any worries they have about whether their child should receive the immunization with the person giving the vaccine.

Reactions to vaccines are unusual and vary considerably in severity. These range from redness and swelling at the site of the injection or a mild fever to excessive crying or a seizure. Medical advice must be sought for serious reactions, and the consequences of further immunizations must be discussed fully before they are undertaken.

Because the infections against which immunizations are available are seen only infrequently these days, a brief word about their signs and symptoms is warranted.

Tetanus is a severe disease causing muscles to contract into painful spasms, and when this disease affects the respiratory muscles it can be fatal. Once the toxin released by the organism has entered the body there is no available treatment. Tetanus is acquired from spores found in the earth, which can enter the body via the smallest cut or scrape. It cannot be passed from person to person.

Poliomyelitis, once commonly known as "infantile paralysis," is caused by a virus that attacks nervous tissue, and it can cause permanent paralysis. If the muscles of respiration are affected, the infection can cause death or require the sufferer to rely on respiratory help throughout his/her life. Milder attacks can occur without paralysis, but in the days before immunization became available the risk of serious handicap or death was always a worrying possibility.

Hemophilus influenzae **type b** (Hib) is an important cause of meningitis in children under the age of 4 years old. Since the introduction of routine immunizations for babies, there has been a marked decline in meningitis due to this cause. (It must be remembered, however, that there are a number of other organisms that can cause meningitis.)

Information about diphtheria, whooping cough, measles, mumps, and rubella can be found in other parts of this volume.

Index